Science, Politics, ...and ME

A health scandal in our generation

IAN GIBSON

ELAINE SHERRIFFS

Copyright © 2017 by Ian Gibson/Elaine Sherriffs

All rights reserved. This book or any portion thereof may not be reproduced or used in any manner whatsoever without the express written permission of the publisher except for the use of brief quotations in a book review or scholarly journal.

First Printing: 2017

ISBN-13:
978-1543183788

ISBN-10:
1543183786

Invest in ME Research

PO Box 561
Eastleigh
Hampshire
SO50 0GQ
UK

www.investinme.org

DEDICATION

To all patients suffering from ME and their families and carers. You have been let down by governments, healthcare departments, the media and by those in positions of influence who could have made a difference but have totally failed you.

Contents

ACKNOWLEDGMENTS vii

About the Authors viii

Foreword xi

Preface xiv

Introduction 1

Chapter 1 – The History of ME 14

Chapter 2   Science and Research 40

Chapter 3 - How the Story Unfolds 74

Chapter 4 - The Politics of it All 94

Chapter 5 –The Biopsychosocial Model 135

Chapter 6 - The Future, not the Past 139

Chapter 7 - Concluding Remarks 160

Appendix 1 - Programme of 11th Invest in ME Research International ME   Conference 2016 166

Appendix 2 – UK Government Ministers of Health 171

Appendix 3 – References 172

ACKNOWLEDGMENTS

Our thanks are due to the following who have aided in our ideas for this book and given up so much time to help their fellow human beings. This all happened when the 'forgotten ones' suffered in silence and occasionally managed to speak out.

    Kevin Short

    Professor Malcolm Hooper

    Dr Dan Peterson

    Associate Professor Mady Hornig

    Dr Nigel Speight

    Richard and Pia Simpson

    Irish ME Trust

    Jon Campling

Not forgetting those carers and ME sufferers, especially Kenny, Karin, Henrik, Ida, Elizabeth, Peter and Ellen who spoke out for us in this book. We hope that their words and our message will bring about action and changes in the attitude to this illness of politicians, scientists and society in general.

Ian Gibson and Elaine Sherriffs

About the Authors

It was whilst Ian Gibson spent a month sitting in Leith's public library, on the edge of Edinburgh, that much of the content of this book took shape. Already Elaine and Ian had met and discussed the book in Norwich, Stockholm and Edinburgh. Both Ian and Elaine knew people whose lives had been devastated by Myalgic Encephalomyelitis (hereafter referred to as ME). Ian is a former MP and Chairman of the UK Government's Science and Technology Committee and has presented at the Invest in ME Research [1] conferences in London since 2006 and chaired them since 2013. Elaine has carried out postgraduate research in both education and anthropology and worked in pastoral care roles for a wide range of young people. However, let's go back to the beginning.

Professor Ian Gibson

This book arose from a challenge by a non-constituent to take ME to be a serious medical problem. My initial reaction was that here was another problem for an MP to either take on or forget. I took it seriously and decided to investigate not by playing the cumbersome role and compelling someone elsewhere to take it up but to do it as a positive mission. My experience had involved cross questioning on a Select Committee of the UK Parliament and many other committees on health and in fact being convinced that Parliament only plays at taking up issues. The more unpopular and difficult ones – the so-called "Too difficult box" are the ones worth getting into. My background in academic research, teaching and cross-

---

[1] Invest in ME are a UK charity nr 1114035- transferring during 2016-17 to CIO charity **Invest in ME Research** (IIMER) charity nr. 1153730

questioning of the 'great and good' sparked the challenge. It is 10 years since we had an inquiry governments have ignored the issue - amongst, of course, many others. These are not only in health but also across the board. Science, in general, and research often seems to elicit a token political response punctuated by the occasional Battle against Cancer initiative of a Vice President. Voices need to speak out and this is our small contribution.

No doubt we shall receive criticism for many different reasons.

BRING IT ON IF IT RECOGNISES THE LIVES OF THOSE QUIETLY SUFFERING AND MISSING OUT ON LIFE.

Elaine Sherriffs

It was whilst working at a university in Norwich from 1991-2008 that I became friends with Ida, a student from Norway, who was physically dynamic and intellectually motivated. She was an undergraduate then postgraduate student who very suddenly, over a period of just a few months, became floored by this little known illness diagnosed as ME. Years of struggle went by and our friendship continued despite her return to Norway and decline in health, but contact became infrequent. Finally, we met again in 2015 and the story of her long illness and slow recovery became an essential component of my involvement in this book. I have before and since met others who have and still suffer from ME. I am sure many, many people reading this book will also know people who have or still have this illness. In fact, it seems to me that everyone knows someone with ME. This makes the importance of this book to raise awareness and urge action to find a cause and cure even more acute.

SCIENCE, POLITICS, …….and ME

Background to the book

At the heart of our work are the voices of the people who suffer the illness, some as patients and others as their carers, and we have interviews with them. It seems appropriate to talk and listen to these people who are not actors but real people. We think this contrasts with the many books on the subject of ME that we have read, and there are many. In particular, we have combed through 'Osler's Web' by Hillary Johnson, Mary Dimmock's book on '30 Years of Disdain', Judy Mikovits and Kent Heckenlively's book 'Plague' and others like Jo Marchant's 'Journey into the Science of the Mind over the Body'.

We do not wish to dwell too much on the past and the 'bad' news, but to describe the new dawn that is opening up in the field of biomedical research into ME. We, of course, have to address the current 'treatments' and ponder on whether the kaleidoscope has truly been shaken and the advent of new approaches will not result in a false dawn.

January 2017

Foreword

From Jon Campling

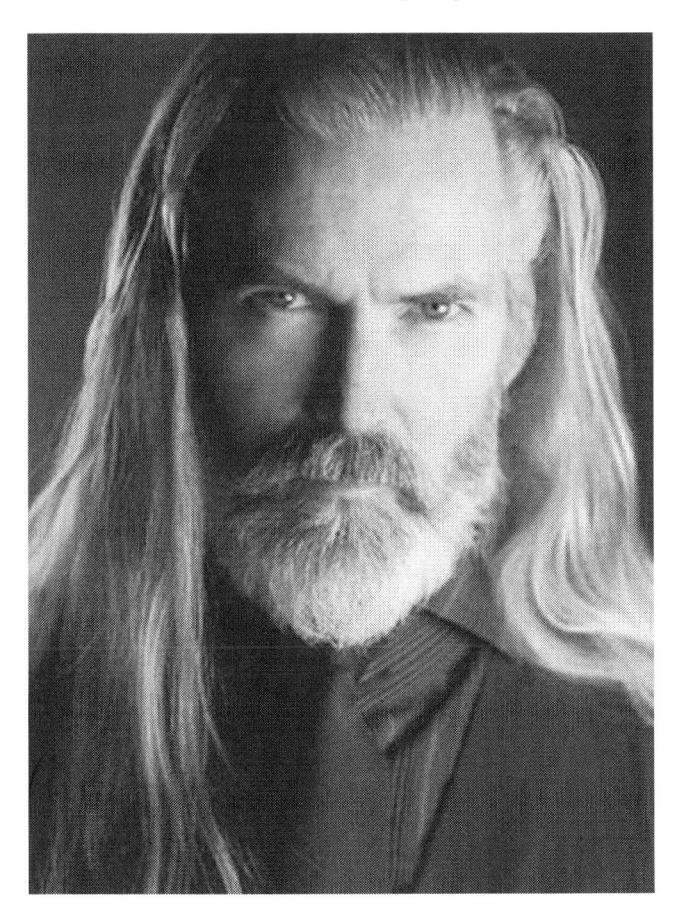

First, let me say how incredibly honoured I was to be approached to provide a foreword to Dr Gibson's book.

For those who do not know me, let me introduce myself. I am an Actor (from Hull), known to many Harry Potter fans as the

'Trainstopping Deatheater', a fierce alias I know, but for me the greatest advantage of that title was the ability to use it to shine my own small but persistent light on the world of ME.

It has helped me start raising funds for Invest in ME Research via my public appearances at many wonderful Comiccons around the country. Having also recently appeared in the latest Final Fantasy release (FFXV) as the powerful but benevolent KING REGIS I hope that too will add to my ability to focus attention and raise funds in the future.

I am married to Ali, who, when we met was also an actor. In fact, she worked far more than I did, being a triple threat (actor-singer-dancer).

With her sights set on the West End she was driven and determined to fulfil the ambition she had held since she was a child. As you can imagine or even have personal experience of, it was heart breaking to see her dream brought to an abrupt halt by this tricksy and incalcitrant illness.

Finally, after 2 years of increasingly debilitating symptoms, she was given a name for her condition - M.E/CFS.

Like those before us, we were soon to realise that with ME the diagnosis is not the beginning of the end as with many illnesses, it does not bring the hope and optimism of a treatment programme that will heal and correct the issue.

Instead, like many, Ali was prescribed 18 months of CBT and advised to use PACING techniques.

We soon realised there was little real understanding of this illness and no ongoing care, so... we found ourselves dealing with it alone, together.

Ali never ceases to amaze me as she deals day in day out with the plethora of ever-fluctuating symptoms whilst always remaining upbeat and positive as she enjoys the life M.E. allows her to have to the fullest.

This book and Dr. Gibson's continued unwavering determination and dedication has, together with an ever-increasing outrage and vocality from the world's estimated 19 Million M.E. sufferers let down by many of the people and organizations that they look to for care, will, I hope, allow M.E. to increase its hard-won momentum towards becoming just another, unremarkable illness.

One that in future medical professionals and the public alike discuss without comment, hesitation or doubt. Accepting fully both its reality and its power to harm.

It has never been more urgent or worthwhile to join together as patients, as carers, as family, as friends to become a force to be reckoned with.

This book is another hard-won step on a long, long journey. A journey so familiar to any long-term M.E. patient and one all newly diagnosed patients come to learn about very quickly.

A journey to undo the mistakes of the past and to look with new eyes, new positivity at ways to understand and one day beat this disease and the damaging misconceptions around it that have challenged us on so many levels and for so long.

The truth is now out, the spirit is still strong and the prize is truly life changing.

Jon Campling January 2017

Preface

Ian Gibson talks to Tom Shakespeare:

During the preparation of this book we have continually wondered why it seems difficult to have support for the funding of biomedical research into ME. Why was the resistance of the medical and legal professions and government departments so consistently strong? We found it hard to believe that a few individuals were able to influence so many people. Influence on policies for the perception, research and treatment of ME seems to have occurred via membership of academic committees, advisory boards of insurance companies, financial resources and the media, in the manner of the establishment. This is not only confined to the field of ME support and research but is the method by which political power is concentrated and enacted. This is how small elites in the UK function and operate.

The anger against those few psychiatrists who seem to be in control has recently been extended to the work on treatments following the large scale funding of the PACE Trial[2] initiative described in Chapter 2. Individuals have retained their academic credibility despite many still feeling their work has been discredited. The psychiatric explanation for ME has been discredited by the recent investigations and questions have been raised in parliament as to whether any fraudulent activity has

---

[2] Comparison of adaptive pacing therapy, cognitive behaviour therapy, graded exercise therapy, and specialist medical care for chronic fatigue syndrome (PACE): a randomised trial White, PD et al. The Lancet, Volume 377, Issue 9768, 823 - 836

occurred in the management of the PACE Trial[3]. The investigation of this government approach has not been acknowledged as yet to be a wrong approach to treatment as with various cognitive therapies. The approach, it is claimed, was another major government supported initiative in which the biomedical approach was ignored.

So I turned to a friend, Professor Tom Shakespeare of the University of East Anglia Medical School, who has studied and published on the subject of disabilities and how political policies are constructed and how these evolve. In particular, he has researched and published work on the biophysical explanation for disabilities and how benefit awards have arisen from the Waddell-Aylward model (see later chapter). This model relates to particular benefits that are based not on biomedical explanations but on social events. As Tom said in our discussion, it relates to causes and it is claimed provides the evidence upon which policy is based. As I show in Chapter 4, it is flimsy evidence which in the case of the causes of ME prevents support for any proposal seeking a biomedical explanation. As he says, when it comes to the award of a benefit (Work Capability Assessment), based on Employment Support Allowance (ESA), there is a not so subtle question asked:

> "Rather than judging whether a person has a practical chance of being able to find a job they can do in the actual labour market, the Work Capability Assessment investigates whether the person has the ability, in theory, to do any form of work at all, thus tightening the eligibility criteria substantially and making it more

---

[3] Written Questions and Answers to Parliament - Written question – 54266 and 54269 http://tinyurl.com/h3rnngq

difficult to qualify for Employment Support Allowance."

Another change has been introduced, as he says:

"A second change is that instead of using a person's regular GP, who knows them and their difficulties, an 'independent assessor' is used, who does not necessarily understand how illness or impairment impacts their life." (Tom Shakespeare)

This can result again in the denial of benefits as we discuss in a later chapter.

Tom based his conclusions on examples of individuals with autism, schizophrenia and dyslexia where studies had centred on bad parenting, headaches and low intelligence without a thorough attempt to seek biomedical factors. He said it was changing significantly, as with ME, as laboratories now sought biomedical explanations. Research was almost certain to unearth the real causes but it was not guaranteed. Evidence using various approaches was necessary but even with a good biomarker for diagnosis a complex situation may unravel a complex interaction between e.g. genes and the environment, including social factors.

Tom emphasised the social class influence on illness and how the environment, both social and physical may lead to successful treatments in one geographical setting and not another. This will predominantly be about environmental differences of housing, food, education, health services and many other factors. But in the life of an individual, living conditions and social class have often been shown to make a similar illness receive different treatments, or even none. Class and health outcomes have been shown time after time to differentiate between people, depending on their class circumstances. This often complicates the attitude of public health servants to provision of a causal understanding where symptoms are complex and treatments are not always 100% successful. There were examples known to him where such discrepancies led to the verdict of the cause of illness as 'we don't know'. This reduces the illness to the 'Too difficult to tackle'.

It sounded like ME was viewed by some as being in this domain.

We agreed that there was much to be angry about in this evidence-based, research-intense country and this included ME.

It meant taking on the elite 'professionals' and challenging their doctrines.

He mentioned the Department for Work and Pensions, the Royal Societies, the Departments of Health, medicine, the media. He has written and spoken of those individuals who hold the purse strings and policy decision-making in their hands.

We agreed we were on our way with an understanding of ME but certain blocks were thrown up by the political parties who failed to take up the question of how to develop better treatments and cures.

SCIENCE, POLITICS, …….and ME

Introduction

This book asks many questions that will challenge governments, scientists and the media. It is a cry for action from 19 million people who suffer in silence from the disease known as ME (also referred to as CFS or ME/CFS) across the world.

The book asks why, over the past 30 years, has there been so little scientific research, treatment or support for the sufferers of the disease known as ME (Myalgic Encephalomyelitis)?

Our purpose is to look at the seeds of change in ME research, particularly at recent developments at the Institute of Food Research (IFR) at the Norwich Research Park supported by the charity Invest in ME Research, where an international centre for research collaboration is being developed. A very small number of research scientists have continued to work relentlessly to find a cause and cure for this condition, swimming against the tide of medical and political bias, often risking professional ex-communication in the process.

One scientist we talked to from the USA has spent many years in the ME field and explained how he leaves any reference to ME off his research grant applications knowing it would receive little sympathetic consideration.

Few politicians have taken any interest. Is this because, unlike HIV/AIDS, it is not perceived to be a fatal disease?

The media have influenced public opinion since the 1980s to believe it is a lifestyle disease resulting from stress, over-activity and an unbalanced life-work ratio. The name Yuppie Flu is thought to have started in the USA and is largely responsible for the disease not being taken seriously for many years. This led to unwillingness by employers, insurance companies, social security and social services departments to treat those suffering from the disease appropriately. Terms such as 'shirker' have also been used. Patients are believed to 'exaggerate' their condition by playing on the illness. The implication is that other patients are serious in terms of talking about their health problems.

Of course, the very symptoms of ME render sufferers incapable of exerting the level of energy required to pursue their cases. The lack of appropriate high quality research and treatment guidelines has left general practitioners and junior doctors with ongoing problems in reaching a correct diagnosis and recommending appropriate treatment for patients presenting with common symptoms.

We do not wish to repeat the individual stories here that have been fully documented in other books and on websites, but we give case studies in order to illustrate important points at the end of some chapters.

Research and treatment

The Medical Research Council (MRC) in the UK, it is believed, have given priority to research funding and political support to the psychiatric route to diagnosis and treatment, at the expense of pursuing the biomedical route involving e.g. immunological considerations. The Gibson Report in 2006 [4] urged the MRC to adopt new approaches to ME research and provide the necessary funds to explore the physiology behind the disease.

In a written request made to the Norfolk and Norwich University Hospital for ME treatments in 2011, the response from the Chief Executive, Anna Dugdale, dated 20 December 2011, stipulated

> "we do not provide a service for ME patients here at the Norfolk and Norwich University Hospital. I believe some confusion may have arisen as our Neurology team have advised

---

[4] http://www.erythos.com/gibsonenquiry/Index.html (2006)

GPs that they see patients with neurological symptoms, as a neurology team they do not see patients without symptoms of this sort".

This comment shows how the official policy of a large university hospital has been to refuse treatment to ME patients on the basis that they did not believe it to be a neurological condition.

The favoured treatments have been psychiatric - Cognitive Behaviour Therapy (CBT) and Graded Exercise Therapy (GET). This is quite incredible and directly contradicts the World Health Organisation (WHO) International Classification of Diseases (ICD). The WHO defines ME under **Neurological Diseases** in ICD 10 section G93.3: Post-viral fatigue syndrome - Benign myalgic encephalomyelitis.

We are astounded that this error of understanding exists at such a senior level of clinical practice and health care management.

Political interventions

One of the authors of this book, Dr Ian Gibson, presented the UK government with a report in 2006 soon after serving as Chair of the Science and Technology Committee under the Labour government (1997-2010). The report was called the 'Inquiry into the status of CFS/M.E. and research into causes and treatment'. It is now 10 years since the Gibson Inquiry was published and little or no action has been taken. The Inquiry recommended that the UK government fund high quality scientific research into the causes and the treatment of CFS/M.E. in contradiction to the Medical Research Council's view that case management and interventions should be the focus. The 2006 Gibson Report summarized the group's recommendations:

This group believes that the MRC should be more open-minded in their evaluation of proposals for biomedical research into

CFS/ME and that, in order to overcome the perception of bias in their decisions, they should assign at least an equivalent amount of funding (£11 million) to biomedical research as they have done to psychosocial research. It can no longer be left in a state of flux and these patients or potential patients should expect a resolution of the problems which only an intense research programme can help resolve. It is an illness whose time has certainly come.

Since that time the MRC have done next to nothing to correct the situation.

Autism and other conditions, for example Alzheimer's, multiple sclerosis and rheumatoid arthritis, have benefited from the more positive campaigns where research has played a major role. Thus 19 million ME sufferers worldwide are still waiting to know the cause of their illness and for an effective treatment to be found.

This book will look at the current situation in the UK and in other countries where again few attempts have been made to progress research. The United States has the largest number of sufferers, an estimated 1 million, but research in the US has been almost entirely funded privately, often by those who have personal experience of relatives or friends with ME and scientists have been challenged, sidelined and sometimes derided for their research. There are signs that the National Institute of Health is now beginning to divert more financial resources into the biomedical research arena. We will describe the extent of this interest in a later chapter. This contrasts strongly with the financial backing given to other issues in society that make it to higher echelons of attention due to high media profile e.g. proton therapy for brain tumours in the recent case of 5-year-old Ashya King, whose parents faced criminal charges for taking their child from a UK hospital to receive proton therapy in the Czech Republic. In 2016, the UK government committed £250 million to developing high-energy proton beam therapy services in the UK and two facilities are currently being built in London and Manchester.

The role of patient support groups

Patient support groups have grown up where governments have failed to act and these organizations join together for conferences, seminars and support new research initiatives. Invest in ME Research hold international conferences with patient groups and internationally recognised experts working on ME such as Hornig, Chia, Baraniuk, Hanson, Davis, Peterson and Kogelnik from the USA, Bergquist and Blomberg from Sweden, Fluge and Mella from Norway, also Marshall-Gradisnik and Staines from Australia, and Scheibenbogen from Germany.

In the UK, we have Cambridge and Bansal in London and Angela Vincent at Oxford, as well as two prominent researchers who are progressing gut research in Norwich, Professors Wileman and Carding based at the University of East Anglia/Institute of Food Research. On and on it now goes with many new names, as shown in the science conference, Biomedical Research into ME Colloquium[5] (BRMEC6), London 2016.

Although patient organisations are active in supporting patients, carers and promoting and financing some research collaborations, they cannot replace mainstream government research funding that will enable scientists to focus exclusively on finding the cause ME and develop treatments. In Sweden, there are 40,000 patients with ME and in Norway 20,000. In Sweden the term "De Osynlinga" (The Invisible Ones) has been used to aptly describe the fate of those with long term and chronic ME

There was a question in the UK parliament by Labour MP Cat Smith on 9 March 2016

---

[5] http://www.investinme.eu/BRMEC%20Colloquiums.shtml#brmec6

"How many GPs have notified cases of ME in the last 5 years?"

In a written reply supplied on 9 March 2016, Jane Ellison, Parliamentary Under-Secretary of State for Health, wrote:

> **This information is not collected in England. The National Institute for Health and Social Care Excellence clinical guidance, Chronic fatigue syndrome/myalgic encephalomyelitis (or encephalopathy): Diagnosis and management of CFS/ME in adults and children, published in 2007, estimates that the annual prevalence is approximately 4,000 cases per million of the population.**

This indicates around 250,000 sufferers in the UK.

The political and scientific background to the inaction surrounding the disease raises many questions that deserve an answer. This book attempts to take an in-depth look at the history of the disease, its misdiagnosis, and the motivation of the main players in the political and scientific arena. At no point should those suffering from this life changing disease be forgotten because it is in their interest alone that this book is written, attempting to throw light on the terrible neglect of their diagnosis, treatment and care endured for far too long.

Throughout many discussions with individuals with muscular and joint pain, as well as fatigue but who remain undiagnosed, similar complaints arise. "It seems to depend on who your GP is when it comes to getting support and a diagnosis' one sufferer commented to me. Several individuals also talk about their children and grandchildren and how difficult it is to lift them up or play with them. Many of them have researched their symptoms online and have a wide understanding and recognize the difficulties of pinning their health problem down to one named condition. This is, of course, due to the overlap of symptoms, e.g. pain or fatigue.

We were impressed by their determination to resist any tendency to become obsessed with their problems. Groups have been set up to allow individuals to share experiences and play a role in their futures. There is a strong belief borne from such discussions that individuals are determined to recover their health.

A feature of many of our interviews was the enthusiasm for participating in clinical trials of treatments and/or treatment with drugs. There was a strong positive commitment for help in the understanding of what causes the health problems by not just contributing financially to research but also to any potential treatments or for anything that improves their quality of life.

Background to ME

Contrary to popular belief, ME is not a new disease but has been documented as far back as 1934 when a mysterious outbreak of debilitating symptoms struck 198 nurses and doctors working at the Los Angeles County Hospital. The symptoms included muscle weakness, instability, cramps and twitches, post-exertion fatigue, neck and back stiffness and sensory disturbances. The illness followed a polio immunization trial of the Brodie vaccine across the US and included staff and children at the Los Angeles County Hospital. The outbreak was described as having symptoms that closely resembled poliomyelitis (polio) but included chronic fatigue. There was some speculation that it was a case of mass hysteria.

The polio virus, now almost entirely eradicated worldwide, is transmitted between humans through faeces or by mouth and occasionally through contaminated water or food. It attacks the nervous system and can lead to muscle paralysis with symptoms such as fever and fatigue, headaches, vomiting, stiffness and pain in the limbs. There is no cure, only prevention through vaccination. The outbreak at Los Angeles General Hospital was believed to be a type of poliomyelitis but the history of the symptoms more closely resembled what we now call M.E.

Other outbreaks resembling poliomyelitis occurred from the 1930s onwards in different parts of the world, Denmark, South Africa, Australia, and in the UK in 1952 in the Middlesex Hospital Nurses Home and 1955 at the Royal Free Hospital. It was here that the name given to this unknown disease for the first time was *benign myalgic encephalomyelitis*.

The epidemics were sometimes considered to be a psychiatric disorder, often misdiagnosed as depression, a misconception that is still common today and the reason for much prejudicial treatment. However, in 1978 the Royal Society of Medicine concluded that ME was a distinct disease with a clear organic basis. Despite this affirmation funding for scientific research did not follow and UK governments continued to pursue psychiatric interventions.

Scientists in the firing line

In the United States a small number of courageous research scientists have pursued the path of a biological cause for the diseases. At the Whittemore Peterson Institute in Nevada, funding for research has been mainly from private sources involving control mechanisms on scientific research which was restrictive and political. Along the way false leads disrupted progress, for example the controversial Xenotropic Murine Leukemia Virus-Related virus (XMRV). This type of research has to take place under extraordinarily complex bio-secure laboratory conditions and the false leads have unfortunately brought scientists such as Dr Judy Mikovits into disrepute.

The ups and downs of scientific research make ME somewhat of a 'hot potato' and it is not a career path that many scientists have been interested in pursuing.

Following the outbreak at Incline Village, Lake Tahoe, Nevada in the mid-1980s a clinic dedicated to treating ME patients was set up by Drs Dan Peterson and Paul Cheney, who have had some success with treatments using both medication and physical therapies. Dr Peterson's clinic in Incline Village, Nevada works in close partnership with Simmaron Research in the same location, on the study of ME. His clinic currently has a waiting list of over 4,000 people. In addition, Dr Peterson travels the world to give talks about his work and research, receiving constant pleas for help wherever he goes from patients seeking a reliable diagnosis and medical treatment. A small number of scientists are involved in research initiatives and remain committed. They attend conferences worldwide that look into the latest research activities and treatments into the disease.

Science is awash with rivalries that contrast with the collaborations. One new area of research is into B cells and other aspects of our immunological system in response to viral infection. Those who are concerned need to map a pathway for reform needed for the revolution into how illnesses like ME are treated. Does it take a czar in each country to effect change or do we need a consortium as is happening currently in Europe? Collaboration can sometimes be substituted by rivalry, as in the case of the contested research findings of Gallo in the USA and Montagnier in France that resulted in long and bitter legal proceedings over the AIDS virus.

Conclusions

This book is therefore timely in its attempt to shake up and alert the political and scientific community to the ongoing suffering of over 19 million people across the world.

The few scientists who are attempting research into the disease struggle to find sufficient funding and are overwhelmed by the pressing needs of patients.

It is time that the 'Invisible Ones' are put into the spotlight and that long overdue answers to their calls for action are given.

To fulfill our task, we reproduce the story of Henrik and his wife who has ME. Henrik is a great campaigner in Sweden and came to the 2016 conference in London.

Case Study: Karin's Journey

'- Hello?
- ...help, help me, can't move... I heard her whisper on the phone. It was December 13th 2009, around noon, and I was having a cup of coffee when the phone rang. It was my wife Karin calling, 25 years old, who was at that time taking a course at the University of Kalmar, 400 km from our home in Stockholm, Sweden. Karin was at the local Ikea store to look for some furniture. As always, she used her bike to get there since she enjoyed the exercise and the cost profile is attractive to a student. After some time at the store she suddenly felt a tremendous exhaustion never felt before together with a burning sensation throughout the body. Her legs could barely support her and she had to lie down on a couch to avoid falling. This was the first sign of ME which, looking back seven years later, still holds her in a firm grip.

Four days prior to the Ikea event, Karin had taken the Swine flu vaccine shot, which the Swedish authorities literally forced everyone to take. The days after the shot the arm was swollen and hurt and she felt a bit like having the flu, but Karin is not the complaining type of person and just continued with the study and other activities waiting for the symptoms to go away.

My initial reaction to her complaints on the phone was "Hey, get up, it cannot be that bad, right?!" After half a minute I realized how bad it was. By a coincidence, my parents happened to be close by Ikea and I called them to pick her up and drive her to the apartment. They helped her in and into the bed, completely exhausted. She was in bed until late the next day, but was still not feeling well. The flu like feeling, exhaustion and legs that could barely move, was still there. After some phone discussions with a nurse, it was decided to take Karin to the hospital since the symptoms were similar to those of the Guillain-Barres syndrome, a life threatening rare condition that also might get triggered by vaccination. In the hospital, they concluded it was not Guillain-Barre but could not give any explanation to the condition and sent her back home.

She still felt something was definitely not right. The following days were spent in bed but as soon as she started to get up all the symptoms came back and lingered for hours: exhaustion, flu like feeling, fever and legs feeling like jelly. The days and weeks passed and the doctors could not explain why the condition did not resolve or why all symptoms worsened after physical activity. Karin finally forced herself to finish the university course with a lot of support from her classmates.

Karin started to work for a company in the food safety business and could just barely work full time. Every weekend she was so exhausted that the whole weekend was spent resting just to be able to go to work Monday morning. Time passed and Karin went in and out of hospital and emergency care since the symptoms got worse and worse over time. No one could explain why. Very few doctors even bothered to perform any deeper examination and concluded *"Your blood tests are within spec, so you can't be ill"*, *"Maybe you're depressed?"* *"Physical activity has never hurt anyone, try harder"* and *"It's so unlikely to get sick from the flu shot so you didn't"*. Karin was forced to change to part time work. The company finally kicked her out since they did not want a sick employee with no diagnosis or future health or work prognosis.

Karin and I got more and more frustrated and started to seek information online and amongst our healthcare employed friends and relatives, but it proved not to be easy. Finally, she met a doctor who almost immediately said "Hey, I recognize this condition, it could be ME!". He arranged further diagnostics to rule out neurological degenerative disorders, sleep disorder, heart and respiratory related disorders etc. All differential diagnostics turned out normal and Karin fulfilled the Canadian ME criteria and finally received a diagnosis, a bit more than a year after the first symptoms emerged.

So, the diagnosis was now a fact, so let's get on with the treatment, right? No. The first thing the doctor said was there is no cure. Not even any proven relieving treatment. The best he could do was start experimenting with any treatments that might at least give a little bit of symptomatic relief.

We realized that Karin had a great bit of luck to meet a doctor that recognized the symptoms and knew about ME. Waiting 10 years or more for a correct ME diagnosis in Sweden is not uncommon.

Karin's condition worsened and worsened. After each physical or cognitive effort, the symptoms flared in what is called Post-exertional malaise. She had to force herself to reduce the activity level to a bare minimum in order not to worsen the condition even further. That involved getting a wheelchair and an electric scooter, reorganize the house to reduce movement and cut down on all unnecessary physical and cognitive activities and instead schedule every day to avoid exceeding the energy expenditure threshold. No more watching TV, meet friends or even sit up while eating. Even with these energy-conserving strategies she continued to get worse and worse.

In the winter of 2011, she was forced to stay all day in bed, except going to the bathroom. She got more and more sensitive to light and noises and had to wear hearing protectors and keep the blinds down during day. She needs help eating, brushing her teeth, change clothes and almost everything else. We have home care support helping her while I am at work. I recently realized how disconnected from the world she was when she asked "Who's Donald Trump?"

Our life plans with kids, nice jobs and an active spare time has been put on hold for an unknown time. For Karin it is a painful standstill where she can only watch the life around her rush by.'

(Our thanks go to Henrik for sharing with us this story of his wife's illness with us).

Chapter 1 – The History of ME

There have been several written accounts of ME, illustrating the problems with medical diagnostics, medical politics and the treatments available to those affected by ME.

There has been a continual dialogue accompanied by lively discussions about the definition of ME. Even to this day there are contentious arguments about the symptoms of ME and the definition.

The lack of universal agreement has contributed to a paralysis of research into causes and this makes it difficult, if not impossible, to get research grants and recognition through peer reviewed research papers. Are similar cases being compared and is it really a heterogeneous collection of individuals being investigated? As we will discuss shortly, the definition of ME being a psychiatric illness and not having a physical cause has been the 'established' position associated with certain individuals who have a direct interest and influence within the political process and with those who make the decisions in government. This opens up funding routes as well as suppressing other views, career progression and leads to the demoralisation of sufferers who have yet to see major progress and discovery.

For too long the battle between individual charities and the official bodies has not led to research discoveries which better lives. It has sometimes spilled over into a vitriolic attack more familiar to politicians and other sectors of public concern.

We believe a more rounded approach to research should be approved. This should be akin to the political approach to the AIDS virus where initial prejudice against certain sectors of our communities by the media and some politicians was replaced with a dramatic injection of finances. One of the authors of this book was telephoned by a senior Cambridge professor from the MRC's (Medical Research Council) molecular biology laboratories and asked to apply for a research grant. It was awarded within days. Very soon basic research increased our understanding of the virus and led to new treatments.

The following statement by the sagacious Professor Malcolm Hooper, University of Sunderland, records the earlier terminology surrounding the illness ME:

> The term Benign Myalgic Encephalomyelitis was first introduced into the UK in 1956 by a former Chief Medical Officer (Sir Donald Acheson) and not by Dr Melvin Ramsay as is sometimes claimed. The word "benign" was used because it was thought at the time that the disorder was not fatal (as poliomyelitis could be, with which it had some similarity), but it was quickly realised by clinicians that ME was not a "benign" condition, as it has such high morbidity (i.e. such a lot of suffering and ill-health), so by 1988 clinicians had stopped using the word "benign" and referred to it as ME, the first to do so being Dr Ramsay. However, the ICD [International Classification of Diseases] still uses the term "benign" in its classification.[6]

In this article Malcolm Hooper defines Benign Myalgic Encephalomyelitis as "a non-fatal disorder (inflammation) of the brain and spinal cord, with pain in the muscles". The ICD (International Classification of Diseases showed that ME was a neurological disorder (1969) and it replaces vague references to mental and behavioural disorders: 'ME cannot be known as or included with neurasthenia or with any mental or behavioural disorder'.

---

[6] http://www.investinme.org/Article%20010-Encephalopathy%20Carruthers.shtml

In the same paper Hooper, who has been a savage critic of any psychiatric explanations of the illness states:

> "It is not true that there is no evidence of inflammation of the brain and spinal cord in ME: there is, but these psychiatrists ignore or deny that evidence."

Hooper also reports that in 1988, in conjunction with the University of Pittsburgh, the US NIAID (National Institute of Allergy and Infectious Diseases) held a large research workshop called 'Consideration of the Design Studies of Chronic Fatigue Syndrome'.

One of the presentations was by Dr Sandra Daugherty, who reported that MRI (magnetic resonance imaging) scans on patients demonstrated abnormalities consistent with demyelination and cerebral oedema in 57% of patients studied. Demyelination is the loss of the protective insulation round nerve fibres, as seen in multiple sclerosis and sometimes also in ME.

Subsequent research involved looking at viral sequences in 1989 and subsequent work through to 1997 involved studies on brain abnormalities, physiology, following post-polio fatigue, viral infections and psychiatric observations of patients. There was an underlying belief around in the research field that differences between the symptoms explained conflicting results. Inflammation of the brain did not appear in patients with chronic fatigue. Neither the 1991 Oxford Criteria, nor the 1994 Centre for Disease Control (CDC) Criteria, were selective of ME patients. They both excluded patients with neurological symptoms or any physical sign of the disease. Further difficulty in progressing research has been associated with a lobby of psychiatrists – collectively known as the

Wessely School[7], who have been known to promote the biopsychosocial model for ME.

The Problems of Definition

There has then been, over some 20 years, a deep-seated argument about the definition or diagnosis of the illness ME.

Clinical practice involves unspecific ailments, alternative pathways, and other competing entities. Severe comorbidities usually overshadow ME symptomology, and there is still no consensus among research groups and health care systems on diagnosis based on clinical criteria. The Fukuda criteria (CDC – 1994) and the Reeves empirical criteria differ in their diagnostic power by a factor of 10. The Canadian Consensus Criteria and the later International Consensus Criteria (ICC) for ME for clinical diagnosis require more specific symptoms. These requirements reflect some current research findings. Major sources of ME cases are those identified by general practitioners (GPs)/family doctors, and neurologists. Smaller numbers are identified by occupational medicine specialists and disability assessors. Paediatric cases are often referred to child psychiatrists. ME still lacks validated molecular diagnostic criteria. (From published data from the distinguished journal, the Lancet, where the work had been subjected to peer review).

In a recent talk on the illness in Stockholm (2015), Professor Leonard Jason of DePaul University in Chicago, USA, who has

---

[7] Hansard reference to the "Wessely School" (Hansard: Lords: 9th December 1998:1013)
http://www.publications.parliament.uk/pa/ld199899/ldhansrd/vo981209/text/81209-07.htm

also been afflicted by ME for a number of years, showed how ME case definitions over the years had shortened, or widened, in the number of individual factors involved in a diagnosis. This made the diagnosis difficult with a uniform series of criteria and still causes much uncertainty about developing a cohort of patients with similar symptoms. Under new proposals from the IOM (Institute of Medicine, USA) the diagnosis of CFS would require 3 core symptoms:

- Fatigue and a reduction in activity that lasts for more than six months.

- Post-exertional malaise.

- Un-refreshing sleep.

In addition, the IOM state that there must be one or other of these symptoms present:

- Cognitive impairment.

- Orthostatic intolerance.

Leonard Jason, who has carried out considerable in depth research into the problems of definition and diagnosis, suggests that those meeting the above criteria vary from 0.4% - 4% of the population. The IOM Committee on Diagnostic Criteria for ME published their paper Beyond Myalgic Encephalomyelitis/Chronic Fatigue Syndrome – Redefining an Illness in February 2015. The IOM report estimates that between 836,000 to 2.5 million people in the USA suffer from this debilitating disorder and that 84-91% of patients affected by the disorder are not yet diagnosed. At the 2015 European ME Research Group (EMERG) meeting [8] in

---

[8] European ME Research Group Meeting http://www.investinme.org/em-index.shtml

London a consensus of opinion was reached to channel research based on the known referral patterns for the disease and share knowledge across scientific strata.

In view of problems with classification and likelihood of subgroups within ME there is a need for infrastructure that will allow mechanistic research to relate back to population-based cohorts and demographic data. ......Long term links between epidemiologists, clinical academics and laboratory researchers need to be secured. [9]

There was, and to some extent there still is, utter confusion due to the different definitions of the condition and conditions. At the above EMERG meeting in London, Professor Jonathan Edwards of University College London, who has widespread experience of rheumatoid arthritis, produced a document with colleagues from Europe that said:

The time has come to develop a co-ordinated programme of biological research into myalgic encephalomyelitis/chronic fatigue syndrome. ME has become the popular way of referring to the illness.[10]

The battle between psychiatrists looking for an explanation in their terms and those looking for biomedical answers in such confusion developed almost naturally, unlike the approach taken with research areas involved in the HIV/AIDS phenomenon. This too, of course, was initially denied by newspapers calling it a 'gay disease or God's wrath', and was accompanied by a campaign to associate the condition with the gay community. This has been shown not just to be prejudicial but also to deny the many other

---

[9] and [5] Jonathan CW Edwards et al *'The Biological Challenge of ME/CFS'*. European ME Research Group (EMERG) Meeting London 13th October 2015

groups of individuals who acquire AIDS (young babies and those receiving blood transfusions).

The scientific community reacted in an inclusive manner and drew in support from many different disciplines. This made it easier for politicians to find the research money and promote widespread investigations. As pointed out in the book 'Plague'[11] by Kent Heckenlively and Judy Mikovits, there were still controversies but some serious scientific investigation led to treatments and political understanding in countries with very different medical treatment models. The approach also drew in the pharmaceutical industries, private and commercial laboratories that also supported further research when drug resistant varieties of the AIDS virus were discovered. Controversy abounded in the USA, and France particularly, over the discovery of this virus by scientists. In the USA, however, a famous top-flight scientist, Peter Duesberg, remained unconvinced of the viral explanation for the AIDS outbreak.

How Scientists Reacted to the Challenges of ME and AIDS

The question arises of how one explanation for causes of ME is favoured and why. Is it for scientific reasons, a hunch, or is there a political bias involving financial or other considerations? Despite the outbreaks of the illness with common symptoms there were many who took that position that hysteria played a major role throughout the years. We have heard of 'copycat diseases', 'flu pandemics', 'AIDS epidemics' etc., all of which are quickly

---

[11] Heckenively K. and Mikovits J. (2014) Plague: One Scientist's Intrepid Search for the Truth about Human Retroviruses and Chronic Fatigue Syndrome (ME/CFS), Autism and Other Diseases. New York: Skyhorse Publishing, Inc.

forgotten, never occurred or were restricted to certain communities.

The association between autism and vaccines was alleged to be evidence-based and even concluded with publication in a peer-reviewed journal. Many children remained unvaccinated and outbreaks of measles occurred. However, the data were flawed and yet the effects of the claim have not yet disappeared in parts of the UK. There is no doubt that the views of professionals are often affected by such events. Indeed, psychological explanations can be favoured in contrast to a biological one, which requires significant finances and serious commitment.

Confusion reigns

The public remained confused or even uninvolved as the debate on ME raged and continues today. Serious discussions were ruled out as scientific bodies ran for cover. There was a serious lack of interest in having open debates at conferences and publicity appeared to be selected by biased individuals or at least on the basis of the view they purported, usually the psychiatric explanation. It certainly wasn't a field of research bursting with ideas and that encouraged new research work or technologies. Scientists no doubt ran for cover into safe subjects for research. The history of today's science still bears the scars of this period through the 1980s to the mid-2000s. It appears to be opening up slowly and new research avenues are being explored. Hopefully the dual hypothesis atmosphere will be eroded and genuine investigations of what causes the illness will now happen.

Meanwhile in the UK, the National Institute for Health and Care Excellence (NICE) produced a rather bland document in 2007 and placed it on a static list in 2014 [this is to be reviewed in 2017[12]]. It gave ME some recognition tackling issues like relapse, diagnosis,

---

[12] https://www.nice.org.uk/guidance/cg53

care and management of the illness. The NICE guidelines were not agreeable to patients though. Supported by most charities patients took NICE to a Judicial Review in opposition to these guidelines [13].

We have yet to meet someone who finds these guidelines useful but at least they are there. They seem to be at some distance from the 2015 Institute of Medicine (IOM) report in the USA but the two committees operated in very different ways. The one in the USA recognised more succinctly the need for research and seemed to believe there would be a solution. The NICE report in the UK does little to help with understanding of the disease and it puts forward little hope for a solution.

Jonathan Edwards, Emeritus Professor of Connective Tissue Medicine at University College London (UCL) has been militating against the lack of research into ME since Invest in ME Research contacted him in order to get him interested in ME research in 2013 -

> [ME] has received almost no attention in terms of research into biological mechanisms. Despite a modest but welcome initiative in the UK by the Medical Research Council (MRC) and hard work by charities, scientific interest in the condition, let alone funding, remains pitifully limited. There may be many reasons for this but there is a growing feeling that it is about time we found a way of addressing this baffling illness in an objective biological framework. Whatever the aetiology, destroyed lives deserve attention.[14]

The introduction of the new diagnostic term, SEID, by the

---

[13] NICE Judicial Review
[14] Jonathan CW Edwards et al *'The Biological Challenge of ME/CFS'*. European ME Research Group (EMERG) Meeting London 13th October 2015

Institute of Medicine in the US brings many issues into contention. "To resolve the "diagnostic impasse" the Institute of Medicine proposes that a new clinical entity, systemic exertion intolerance disease (SEID), should replace the clinical entities ME and CFS. However, adopting SEID and its defining symptoms, does not resolve methodological and diagnostic issues. Firstly, a new diagnostic entity cannot replace two distinct, partially overlapping, clinical entities such as ME and CFS. Secondly, due to the nature of the diagnostic criteria, the employment of self-report, and the lack of criteria to exclude patients with other conditions, the SEID criteria seem to select an even more heterogeneous patient population, causing additional diagnostic confusion."[15]

The Cost of ME to Society

The IOM Committee in the USA estimates that the direct and indirect costs of ME to society are between $17 and $24 billion annually. Leonard Jason predicts that with the name change for the disorder to SEID (Systemic Exertion Intolerance Disease) and with the new clinical definition, a much larger cohort of patients will be included in SEID statistics drawing from those patients who are currently diagnosed with either depression or a physical illness with similar symptoms to ME.

We will mention more recent attempts to tackle the problems around ME e.g. definition, treatment etc., here in the UK and in other countries, like the USA. It is an international field of interest and maybe this in itself deserves an international, global approach for tackling the problems. This seems a long distance away at this time. 250,000 people within the UK and 49,000 in Sweden seem destined to remain dissatisfied with the current knowledge of the illness and frustrated by the lack of treatment. As one major player

---

[15] Twisk, F.N. Replacing Myalgic Encephalomyelitis and Chronic Fatigue Syndrome with Systemic Exertion Intolerance Disease Is Not the Way forward. *Diagnostics* 2016, 6, 10.

in research from a major centre in the USA said at a recent conference, "unless you undertake some treatment in the first 6 months, it is then too late". The cost has been estimated in the UK as £3.5 billion [16]annually in medical services, social benefits and lost incomes to individuals. In the USA it is $9.1 billion in lost productivity on top of medical cost and disability payments. Families lose $20,000 income a year due to ME in the USA.

The Conflicts in Science

About the same time at a Stockholm conference in October 2015 a meeting in England of different researchers (EMERG) from European countries concluded

A strength of the ME community is intense discussion of potential biological mechanisms, drawing on an informed but sceptical perspective, between individuals with expertise in different disciplines, bringing together laboratory scientists, patients and carers.[17]

Of course, there are the two competing groups of researchers who some feel may be subsuming their differences as they search for the causes. One thing is clear, whether you believe ME is best represented to the public as myalgic encephalomyelitis, a post viral syndrome or chronic fatigue immune dysfunction syndrome, people are affected by post-exertional malaise, impaired muscles or joints, irregular sleep, gastric problems, memory loss and poor concentration, as the common features.

In a large number of cases the commencement of problems is

---

[16] From Sheffield Hallam University report published in 2003
http://news.bbc.co.uk/1/hi/health/3014341.stm

[17] Jonathan CW Edwards et al *'The Biological Challenge of ME/CFS'*. European ME Research Group (EMERG) Meeting London 13th October 2015

linked to a viral infection but other sufferers may have the onset linked to an operation or accident. Many are experiencing the onset of common symptoms as a slower process whereas others report sudden and distinct onset, as illustrated in the interviews with sufferers which we have recorded in this book. This can affect both employment and education, both of which are difficult if not impossible to sustain when suffering from ME. Social pastimes and activities within and outside families are extremely limited. Many people remain bed or house bound for months, if not years, as witnessed in our interviews. Whole families are affected by this disease.

Case Study: Ellen

Ellen was a busy, active happily married thirty-six-year-old mother of three who worked full time as a senior healthcare assistant in a residential home for the elderly.

> I can remember the day that I first became ill. It was mid October 1993 and we were enjoying a lovely Indian summer, the weather was roasting and I was looking forward to finishing my shift and taking the kids to the beach for a couple of hours after school. We came home from the beach about 6.30pm and I felt a bit unwell as if I had a cold coming and decided that once the kids' homework and baths were done and next day's lunches prepared that I would have an early night.

> I felt so ill the next morning that I couldn't go to work, it seemed to me like the worse flu I had ever experienced. I couldn't lift my head, my neck was so sore and the light hurt my eyes, I just wanted to sleep. My husband wanted to call the GP out but I told him it was just flu and that I would be over it soon. I was in bed for a few days and then eventually made it downstairs. Although I was feeling a bit better I was still far

from well. After ten days I returned to work, convincing myself that I just needed to shake it off. I was only back in work two days and I had to stay off again. This became the pattern for the next fifteen months. I used to feel awful having to inform my boss that I wouldn't be in work yet again. I was brought up to work hard, my parents always told us that hard work didn't kill anyone so I was constantly telling myself to buck up.

I started to experience a whole range of strange symptoms. One morning as I tried to get out of bed my legs wouldn't work, they just went from under me and I couldn't stand or get back on the bed for twenty minutes, this happened on a couple of occasions whilst I was at work. I seemed to have a continual cold, I kept getting chest and ear infections. I had the most excruciating muscle spasms in my legs and pins and needles in my feet and hands and with each week I became more and more exhausted. Each week I thought if I can just have a few days' rest I will be better by next week, or then the next or by summer or Christmas and so on it went. I just couldn't understand what was the matter with me, why I felt so ill, weak and exhausted. I was becoming very forgetful; it was like I couldn't get my brain to work properly. I couldn't spell the simplest of words and sometimes I couldn't remember how to form the letters that spelt my own name, sometimes I couldn't remember my name, on a number of occasion's at the supermarket checkout, I would need to check my name on my debit card before I could sign the receipt. It seemed like overnight I couldn't do the simplest of additions. I couldn't count my change correctly to tender my bus fare or work out how much money for the school lunches. I became confused at road crossings and would think that the red light meant go and the green stop. I seemed to lose half of my vocabulary too.

Things were just getting worse at work as I had become so unreliable so I dropped down to three days a week. I returned to work after ten days off determined that I would be able to manage my three shifts for that week. I went to work one morning January 1995 feeling even more dreadful than usual, I collapsed that day in work with severe chest pains, a colleague caught me as I fainted.

I can remember feeling very cold but my colleague later remarked that she had never seen such an awful pallor or known anyone to radiate such heat from their head and body. This was fifteen months from my initial illness. I have been unable to work since.

My boss called my GP who assured me that I wasn't having a heart attack and asked if I wanted him to admit me to hospital. I didn't want to go to hospital so my GP advised that my boss take me home and for me to go straight to bed. My GP visited me at home about an hour later, again he assured me again that it wasn't my heart but he said he wasn't really sure what was the matter with me. He said that he feared admitting me to hospital as wards were being closed due to various outbreaks in local hospitals and that I could catch something else to complicate things. I trusted my GP, had he thought that I needed to be in hospital he wouldn't have given me any choice in the matter, he did insist though that I stay in bed. I can't remember much about the next couple of weeks but my GP came in most days at all sorts of odd hours. One day he arranged for a consultant physician from the local hospital to visit me home, the consultant agreed with the GP that I was very poorly and better off at home rather than in hospital but he had no idea what was the matter with me. He did an ECG at home but wanted to do x-rays and a scan and arranged for a car to pick me up and take me to the hospital forty miles away. I was eventually diagnosed with Bornholm's Disease; it seems there was an outbreak of this in the area that month.

I improved slightly but most of the time was a blur of pain, nausea and exhaustion. I had awful sinus infections that were incredibly painful and I felt extremely ill with the least exertion. One day I realised that I couldn't see properly to read a letter and I made an appointment with the optician. The optician started to examine my eyes and suddenly asked if I was in poor health. She went out of the room and phoned my GP and by the time I arrived home from the opticians the local hospital has phoned to say that I had an emergency appointment with a neurologist for the next day. It seems that the optician had noticed white patches in the back of my eyes and was quite concerned. The neurologist sent me for some tests, when I went back to see him he said there was nothing wrong and I was probably depressed.

At best I was functioning at below thirty percent of what I normally did but more often I could just about manage to get to the bathroom, I couldn't bathe or shower without assistance. At my worst I couldn't ask for a drink if I was thirsty or if I was brought one I didn't have the energy to sit up to reach over to pick the glass up, I couldn't even ask for help to have the drink. If my duvet fell off I couldn't pull it back on again but had to wait until someone looked in the room and see that I was lying there cold. I often couldn't move or adjust my position in attempt to make myself more comfortable. The slightest movement from the chair or bed if somebody brushed past used to cause me awful motion sickness and painful jerks in my legs. The only relief I could get from this was to lay perfectly still on a duvet placed on the floor.

My GP was very good and continued to try to find out what was the matter with me, he was as puzzled as I by some of the new symptoms that kept appearing, a dozen or so small lesions started to appear on my hands, I had a strange red rash on my neck and jawline, I often had no feeling in my thumb and fingertips, I had shooting pains in my skull and agonising pains shooting up through the soles of my feet that could send me sprawling. Some people had started to suggest that maybe I had ME, I mentioned this to the GP but he said he wasn't convinced. The GP said that he was very disappointed with the attitude of the neurologist and referred me back to the consultant physician who had visited me at home, my GP was about to retire and he said that he wanted me sorted before he left.

The consultant asked me to list my symptoms, severity etc., he said that MS and Lupus had been ruled out by other consultants. I asked him about ME and he said that he didn't know much about it, he gave me an appointment for the following week. At the next appointment he said that he had done a bit of reading about "this ME" and that he had arranged for me to have a SPECT scan later that week.

When I went for the scan the technician jokingly asked did I have friends in high places at the hospital because they only did two SPECT scans a year as they were so expensive.

When I saw the consultant at my next appointment, he said that the bad flu I had described from eighteen months earlier had been Encephalitis, he said that I had severe scarring and lesions on the left temporal lobe of my brain and a reduced blood flow. He said that I was now the first person he had ever diagnosed with Myalgic Encephalomyelitis and it was not CFS (but at that time I didn't understand what he meant) He said that he believed that I could get better but it would take three, four or even more years, he told me to go away and find out as much information about ME that I could and he would do the same and that he would see me again in six months to discuss what we would do. Unfortunately, the consultant was away ill at my next appointment and I was rather bewildered when his replacement said that he didn't want to talk about that ME nonsense, he was only interested in the rash on my neck and jawline. I was given another appointment to see my regular consultant but due to moving house 200 miles away I was never able to see him again.

Unfortunately, I have never had the same level of care or interest from a GP or consultant since then, quite the reverse in fact. I honestly believe that my last GP has been deliberately unhelpful and dishonest about referral letters and other requests for help but I was just too ill and let things slip and maybe too scared of the GP. I'm not a timid person and have never been afraid to fight or speak up for what I believe in but I now find it hard to do so for myself when it comes to ME. When I first started to read up about ME I read a lot of bad patient experiences about the medical profession and how many people with ME (pwme) are treated badly by them. I couldn't understand that, as that was certainly not the way I had been treated. But fast forward a couple of years and sadly I found out for myself what exactly most pwme were complaining about.

I did start to develop cardiac problems and was taken to hospital a few times with either excruciating chest pain or severe tachycardia. I know that the staff were concerned and insisted that I be admitted to the cardiac ward. A few causes for the chest pain were suggested, angina, arterial spasms, pleurisy. Unfortunately, once the cardiac consultant became aware of the ME diagnosis he became very rude and patronising and I was never properly investigated. I was dismissed with "you CF (chronic fatigue) patients are all the same".

I could see the shock on the ward sister's face at how this consultant was behaving towards me. After one admission to hospital I was given angiogram, the report sent to my GP stated that the arteries were clear however I had had an arterial spasm whilst undergoing the procedure. I told the GP this had been suggested for earlier and ongoing bouts of agonizing chest pain but he dismissed it by saying it was of no consequence and didn't need further investigation/treatment. Once, whilst in hospital, I could hear a nurse outside my cubicle arguing with the doctor about me, she was saying that it was obvious that I was very ill and that I needed to be admitted but the doctor just shouted her down. Before I left the nurse advised me to take the doctors name and make a complaint, she said that I was very poorly and shouldn't be getting treated this way. As I was leaving the ward another nurse started to call my name and told me to get back into bed at once, when I told her that I had just been discharged she insisted that I sit right down and wait while she checked to see what was going on, when she returned I could see that she was bemused too but she just shrugged and apologised.

Some doctors that I've seen over the years about non-ME related problems have tried to be helpful, when they detect something is not quite right. I had surgery for a detached retina a few years back and had to return to the hospital for a follow up the next day. I was feeling quite unwell with the ME and suddenly fainted, each time I came to and the nurses tried to sit me up I would faint again. It was nearly an hour before I could get up to see the consultant, who remarked on how very ill I looked and asked what treatment was I receiving for my shocking blood pressure. I told him I wasn't receiving anything and he advised that I see my GP asap, then he added "you poor ME patients get a rough deal don't you?" When I did get to see my GP he dismissed it (without even taking my BP) as stress at being in a hospital waiting room.

I started to develop allergic type symptoms, bouts of sneezing, persistent coughing, streaming eyes etc. I became very ill if I took antihistamines in an effort to relieve the symptoms. I asked my GP if I could have allergy testing in an effort to ascertain what I was reacting to but he wouldn't hear of it. Eventually things got so bad that I couldn't breathe properly due to nasal polyps and he eventually referred me to ENT. The consultant there was shocked when he examined me and asked why I waited so long to get referred... he said that he needed to establish just what I was allergic to and we must start by ordering IgE blood tests. Unfortunately, it was a different consultant at the next appointment who said there was no need for that and wouldn't allow me to have a copy of the results. He maintained that if I knew the results I would make myself live in a glass bubble....

I expect like everyone else who has to claim sickness benefits, I live in dread of the renewal forms and medicals required to continue being paid ESA etc. but every doctor that I have seen at these assessments have acknowledged that I'm very ill. One doctor actually apologised to me for having to attend the medical centre, the assessment took less than five minutes and he advised me to go home and call my GP out to the house as I was very poorly. A few years later I was called for another medical. I didn't recognise the doctor but he explained that he was the same doctor from my previous assessment. Again he was very quick and apologetic, he said that he was annoyed as he had written on my file at my last visit that I wasn't to be called again.

I hate this illness, it's had a massive impact on my family, bad enough that I was unable to work and help provide for my family but I could no longer care for them, they were having to care for me. Everything started to revolve around me and my needs. Not only were my husband and children having to cope with caring for me and all that running a home entails, they also had to do a lot for my mum too. The thing I really hate was how my illness dictated what they could and couldn't do, not only had my freedom been curtailed but so had theirs, simple things like them not being able to play their music because of the noise making me ill and having to have the lights dimmed. I felt like a killjoy as if I was always moaning, turn the music down or lights off, don't use that deodorant or that perfume etc. etc. The kids hated that I was always too ill for even simple things like a walk down to the seafront to buy ice creams after tea. I couldn't get to their activities such as football matches and school plays and concerts. Holidays and day trips were out of the question. Trips to the nearest beach when I could make it out were often cut short because I would start to feel ill and need to come home or would take me weeks to recover from. I felt so guilty at not being able to give my family the care and attention that I wanted to, it felt bad not being able to give my mum the support and care that she deserved. It was awful having to miss out on family and friends' occasion's such as weddings and other important events. I was even too ill to travel to attend my father's funeral.

I stopped thinking that I would be better by next week but I was convinced that it was only a matter of time, like next year or the year after…I try not to think of all things that I've been unable to do since becoming ill, the plans we had for ours and the children's lives, the longed for travel with and when they were older without our kids. I hate how I just can't be spontaneous and suddenly decide to even jump on a bus and go exploring. It's simple things I really miss, like not having the radio on constantly at home and singing (badly) along to the music or if a particular favourite comes on dancing (very badly) around the room.

I'm embarrassed to have to claim benefits and to have not been able to make provision for my old age, to no longer have savings etc. When I do meet up with siblings, family members or old friends I'm not so bothered when they speak of their holidays and travels, new houses and kitchen extensions etc. but I dread the conversation turning towards jobs, careers, pensions etc. or when I meet new people and they ask what I do, It's not as if I have been feckless or lazy, just ill.

I'm fully aware that I'm not as badly affected by this awful disease as some are and I'm truly thankful for that. I've had some pretty bad crashes in the past and dread it happening again. I can only imagine how it must be for the very severely affected or those without the love and support from family or friends. I do class myself as one of the luckier ME patients in as much as although ME has spoilt things for me I did have a life before ME, unlike the children and young people who have ME. No matter how ill I've been I'm always thankful that it's me and not my kids who have it. I feel lucky that I had my children before I was ill, I'm now a grandmother but many of my fellow ME patients (and their carers) have been denied their chance of children and grandchildren of their own. They didn't actually choose this, having ME made that decision.

(Our thanks go to Ellen – not real name - for sharing her story with us)

Research is essential to find a way forward, and especially the biomedical approach looking for biological/medical pointers.

'ME can be beaten by taking more exercise and positive thinking', landmark study claims'. [18]
This headline in the Mail Online was seductive in 2015, except this was not the conclusion of the work by the Oxford psychiatrist, Professor Michael Sharpe, when a few hours later he appeared on a

---

[18] MailOnline www.dailymail.co.uk/health/article-3292782 28 October 2015

BBC programme. The article claimed that sufferers of ME or Chronic Fatigue Syndrome did not push themselves to recover. The debate between those who supported a psychiatric explanation of the condition or those who believed its explanation lay in physiological events was renewed once more. Cognitive Behavioural Therapy (CBT) would overcome fears of taking exercise. The UK government had made a large financial commitment to this therapy during the Labour administration under Tony Blair.

The Establishment Wakes Up

The evidence of a concerted media campaign to extol the virtues of the psychological approach is clear from the work of the Science Media Centre in London. The origins of this initiative I remember well. Discussions over breakfasts in the Royal Institution in London brought about its birth and it has developed over the years from the early 'noughties' to the 21st Century. Its aim was to aid a wider understanding of science in the population but also to affect an understanding of the work carried out in the laboratory within the House of Commons and Lords. Almost in parallel, a group called 'Sense about Science' was set up by Lord Taverne and with a fair degree of success presented scientific personnel to explain the evidence. Recently a debate on ME on radio had Professor Simon Wessley as its expert. Too often alternative views are referred to as 'quackery.' The recognition that Science thrives on controversy is replaced by a too often 'there is only one answer'. The evidence is overwhelming, so just listen to the expert!!

We will discuss the current thinking and the scientific evidence for causes, cures and alleviations of the symptoms in Chapter 2. However, suffice it to say at this point that the issue of ME, its origin and treatments, surfaces at regular annual periods in all countries, which the authors have visited. Certain universities have teamed up in the UK to maintain a perception of the disease as being predominantly found in a certain social class and it is seen as not a serious worry for conventional medicine.

Recently a campaigner from a mental health campaign group berated one of the authors of this book about ME being a 'middle class problem'. Efforts to address the problem centred on the PACE Trial (Pacing, graded Activity, and Cognitive behaviour therapy; a randomised Evaluation) research into ME, which is described in a later chapter, has come in for much criticism. Even Climate Change scientists who have argued for serious political activity to reduce serious effects in both the short term and long term, have come to realise that pillorying the opposition is not the way to handle the issue. Calling ME 'yuppie flu' seeks to ridicule the serious problems. It was clear people were ill and just because there is no clear definition or agreement this should not prevent serious research. In the UK questions were asked in both Houses of Parliament - the Countess of Mar in the House of Lords and others in the Commons - where the issue was dismissed. It seemed governments everywhere played it down. The polarisation of the debate around the causes of ME and even the definition and diagnosis of the illness ensured the press would take a low profile. There were no major headlines as with AIDS, but there were articles about malingerers and skivers.

Patient Support Groups

We have made it a central theme to talk to patients and their support organisations. Without an appreciation of the lives they lead, the problems they suffer and how their lives and families and friends are often on hold, we miss the essential problems that need addressing. We are aware of the work with other conditions, some of which have been incorporated into the medical programmes of ME. Cancer research is held up as the standard at which to aim. However, it should be noted that cancer research is co-funded to a large extent by charity money. We will illustrate at appropriate points in our analysis of advances in Multiple Sclerosis, Parkinson's Disease, autism and dementia and rheumatoid arthritis to convince the reader that a combined political and scientific approach can lead to advances for the benefit of patients. ME research still lags behind and we will illustrate this point from different countries and within a country. Charities, too, can behave in different ways across borders, depending on the political environment – or even within the same country.

Nevertheless, research is taking place with new approaches that are gradually being recognised. However, governments e.g. in the UK, favour the psychiatric approach and this is mainly shown through the established research committees and politicians involving both personalised and institutionalised mechanisms. The names of the same individuals appear in Dept. of Health Committees and on many other bodies with control over research grants and policy forming bodies. There is however, through the work of various charities and research for a scientific understanding, a new wave of enlightenment on the horizon, and the process of crowd funding has started in the ME field to resource the necessary finances.

The ME Patients

How do patients deal with this disease? After various lengths of time individuals may return to a better cycle of health. These are few in number but in this category the majority of individuals live a day-to-day, or month-to-month existence with good days and bad. Any relapse period can be exacerbated by infections, stress, operations etc. We find that many are severely affected and need practical and social support. A significant few continue to deteriorate in their health and require medical support and further diagnosis.

Case Study: Elizabeth

I met Elizabeth in Scotland in early 2016. It is 11 years now since the initial onset of the symptoms corresponding to ME. The first sign of illness came after a time of two bereavements, the sale of her family home followed by a house move and years of renovating an old property. These were traumatic and exhausting life events for Elizabeth and although she had asthma as an underlying health problem she had no other disease, virus or illness at the time. The first sign of something more seriously wrong was the onset of breathing problems that were initially put down to asthma, "I just couldn't breathe at all, I was gasping"

Her GP prescribed steroids but this had no effect. A specialist at the regional hospital in Scotland examined her but concluded that it was possibly depression and Elizabeth was then referred to a psychologist who prescribed CBT. At the same time she carried out a self-test of cortisone levels and she found she was flat lining. With a background of working in the NHS she had read about adrenal fatigue and so started to work on nutrition as a way of restoring her health, drawing information from the writings of the nutritionist Gillian McKeith. Within a period of months she suffered a series of dramatic physical collapses.

> "One day I was gardening and suddenly found I couldn't walk, I was on my hands and knees". Another time she was in a supermarket and found that "my legs just turned to jelly. I couldn't stand or walk".

> Throughout all this time Elizabeth continued to work but found it more and more difficult to maintain the daily routine, so eventually changed to part time work. This change of job caused a lot of stress and brought on a mental and physical shut down. She felt confused and depleted and

now, 11 years on, the first signs of stress or overwork bring back all physical and psychological problems. Her health has become extremely vulnerable to any overload. She has occasional inflammations, fatigue and breathing problems, but says "I consider myself lucky compared to many others with ME"

There are people she has met though a support group who have been ill for up to twenty years and in some cases have lost their careers, their partners and their mobility. Elizabeth and other members of the group have applied for social security benefits related to their illness (Employment and Support Allowance, which replaced Incapacity Benefit in 2008), but have been refused benefits on the basis that ME is not considered a long term illness that prevents people from being employed on a full or part time basis. The whole process of applying for and being refused benefit for the illness was very distressing – more on this in Chapter 3.

When applying for jobs Elizabeth kept quiet about her ME for fear that it would be misunderstood or held against her in future employment. Indeed, when she fell ill the first time her manager advised her to resign without mentioning the real reason (ME) for leaving, knowing that future employers might be prejudiced against her. Elizabeth does fear other people's reactions and assumptions. The disease has changed her life and the prospect of a relapse is a constant threat ["I have had to adjust all my expectations of myself"] as though she has a continual sense of doom hanging over her.

(Our thanks go to Elizabeth – not real name - for sharing her story with us)

Chapter 2   Science and Research

1. Past Directions

The problems of understanding the illness

As we researched this book we have continually been drawn into the concerns about a definition of the condition(s) and at the same time the two major groupings on how to provide treatment, psychiatric or physiological. There is of course a school of thought that thinks both factors are involved and exploring one or other is a deliberate ploy to confuse and obscure the issue. We have met academics, scientists, medical doctors, politicians and individuals who think there is no such condition, even suggesting it is a 'skivers' character or 'middle class' angst. It was interesting how little many individuals had heard of ME through their professional training as medical students. We will show how the charity Invest in ME Research has developed support for research often against the professional grain to produce research at the university in Norwich and publicise their findings in the press. There is a huge amount of literature in this field but little explaining how and why the medical and political establishment resist progress in the field of biomedicine favouring instead the psychosocial approach. We will attempt to explore why this is prevalent across countries and how political action and new scientific initiatives are essential to 'redress the crimes'.

Like ME, illnesses such as autism and dementia were at one time ignored and some would say the same was true of Rheumatoid Arthritis, Lupus, Multiple Sclerosis, Parkinson's, Muscular Dystrophy etc. etc. etc. During the Blair years of government cancer research and treatment became a priority and also mental health. Over the course of the period 1997-2010 both cancer and mental health were given large financial sums and there were improvements to services. These have now slipped back and it is

1997 again with the National Health Service in dire trouble. Patients are suffering long waits, treatments are denied, and private facilities are taking over care of patients and treating of illnesses. Services are being reduced within the NHS and facilities are not responding to the numbers of elderly patients in the community. There have been some glimmers of hope. Other illnesses are being tackled with a different emphasis and this is having reverberations in the ME world. The beginnings of a political campaign across Europe for ME biomedical research is gaining support. We will concentrate on the situation in Norwich and how we are progressing a research programme after a long campaign. This will involve the research at the University of East Anglia and the Institute of Food Research in the UK.

First, however, in the recent book by Steve Silberman 'Neurotribes'[19], the history of autism is recounted. The description of autism in children involved on the one hand describing them as "socially awkward, had precocious abilities and fascination with rules, laws and schedules" and on the other hand others describing them as "low functioning children" caused by bad parenting. This latter view was the preferred view of the medical establishment. In the 1990s onwards the diagnosis changed to that of autism being on a 'spectrum', a continuum with different degrees of severity. Questions have been raised involving explanations of MMR vaccines for Measles, Mumps and Rubella, causing autism and solutions might be as simple as no vaccination against these diseases or treatment with vitamins. Major events, however, which raised the doubts about the earlier explanation of autism, were brought about with the film 'Rain Man' starring a sympathetic actor, Dustin Hoffman, who portrayed the life of one autistic individual. This is an example of the influence of celebrities.

---

[19] Silberman, Steve (2015). 'Neurotribes: The Legacy of Autism and How to Think Smarter About People Who Think Differently'. London: Allen and Unwin.

The words and language used in illness were always political which bears similarity to the history (until now) of ME. Even the diagnosis has political connotations. As a reviewer has said "it is only being identified as a disorder, described in diagnostic manuals so that one can access the educational and other services that some autistic people require to flourish" (Silberman, 2015). Many case studies suggest the same storyline with ME. The search for a simple definition fails to recognise that individuals are just that. They can each have a different combination of symptoms. Phrases like neurological and neurodiversity must be considered and this reveals that one area of the medical profession is often too rigid in demanding precise definitions. This may even mean that there is no one biological marker in every illness in the face of its heterogeneity. It may mean several markers are needed to aid identification. This is also as true in cancer as in autism.

To progress the case of understanding the current situation regarding ME research and treatment this chapter will give an overview of the various research initiatives followed in different countries and the results so far. The path to diagnosis and treatment has been littered with controversies involving professional rivalries, financial and political restraints, reputations and careers that have been ruined. The political influences here, in our view, have been paramount. We have recently been in touch with many scientists who are unravelling the chemical and brain pattern changes in ME patients. The new wave of enthusiasm over early biomarkers and causes may some day be unveiled as the research field moves on. This will, of course, require a political response by funding bodies or governments.

Clinical Research Centres

There are several centres of research across the world. CII at Columbia University in New York, Center for Enervating

NeuroImmune Disease at Cornell University in Ithaca, The Nevada Center for Biomedical Research (formerly the Whittemore Peterson Institute) in Nevada, the Simmaron Institute also in Nevada, Stanford ME/CFS Initiative, Open Medicine Institute in California, Institute for Neuro Immune Medicine in Florida, Bateman Horne Center in Utah, National Centre for Neuroimmunology and Emerging Diseases (NCNED) in Australia and others are now set up or setting up in Sweden, Germany, Norway and Japan. Since most of these are interested in physiological explanations they try to treat patients as best as they can whilst research progresses.

In the UK the new kid on the block is Norwich where the Centre of Excellence is undertaking research into the gut microbiome, similar to research in New York and Cornell in the USA.

It is very early days yet but the team of interested research collaborators is growing.

Funding of Research

In the UK both biomedical and psychological research is receiving funding now and groups can be found in Newcastle, Bristol, London (UCL and Kings College) and Oxford, as well as Norwich. The sources of funding are the Medical Research Council (MRC) in the UK and the crowd funding by charities like Invest in ME Research. In the States the National Institute of Health (NIH) has invested over the last year some funding to complement that from private sources.

At the 2016 Invest in ME Research Conference in London the NIH spokesperson pointed out the huge disparities in award for Lupus research in contrast with ME (see later).

The under-funding is even starker when the prevalence is

considered. According to an analysis done by Dr Andreas Kogelnik, ME clinician and founder of the Open Medicine Institute in the USA, the per-patient funding level for this disease is less than any other disease and far below that of other diseases of similar prevalence and/or morbidity. For instance, annual funding for this disease is about five dollars per patient, whole that for multiple sclerosis is about $255 per patient and HIV/AIDS is about $2,482 per patient. To be equitable based on disease burden and prevalence, ME funding would have to be roughly $250 million a year......This low level of research funding is not an historical anomaly. Since the inception of NIH's ME program in about 1987, NIH funding for this disease has never been higher than $7.2 million (in 2002) and averaged about $5.0 million since 1987. The change in the NIH budget for CFS from 1995 to 2014 represents a decrease of about 27 per cent at a time when total NIH funding increased about 166%.[20]

Stumbling Progress

Progress towards isolating a biomarker continues, haunted by a history of controversy and false leads and plagued by disproportionate lack of research funding for such a serious disease. The much publicised trial of scientist Judy Mikovits, once a leading light in the pursuit of ME research, demonstrates the minefield discovered by scientists entering this field of science. The XMRV (Xenotropic Murine Leukemia Virus) research carried out by Mikovits at the Whittemore Peterson Institute for Neuro-Immune Disease laboratory in Nevada was discredited in 2012 following contamination of human tissue with mouse viral nucleic acid sequences present in the laboratory samples. The retrovirus was believed to be a contributing factor to Chronic Fatigue Syndrome. The book 'Plague' written by Mikovits and

---

[20] Dimmock M and Lazell Fairman M (2015) *Thirty Years of Disdain: How HHS buried ME*. Available online: http://bit.ly/The_Burial_of_ME_Background

Heckenlively, referred to in Chapter 1, describes the internecine warfare that took place amongst scientists, editors of medical journals and those individuals and institutions funding research, all desperate to be the first to find the root cause of and successful treatment for ME. The excitement over the 'discovery' has now subsided but the wounds of research scientists have been slower to heal. Again, the story is one of rivalry, spin doctoring, malicious gossip and competition rather than collaboration. Prominent researchers and politicians in Washington were drawn into a world of subterfuge, spin and nasty rivalries.

Therapeutic treatments

The first therapeutic trial for ME was undertaken by Max Allan Banfield in Australia, a gymnast who, after suffering from CFS at the age of 25, developed the idea of pacing himself through physical exercises over a period of 12+ weeks supported by a medical research team including two research cardiologists and a laboratory with the latest medical technology to monitor the progress of clients. The exercise programme he designed was submitted as an article to the BMJ in 1982 with reference to studying the effects of regular exercise on CFS. The BMJ finally published his study in 2013.[21]

Behavioural therapies such as CBT and GET have been considered by some as an effective treatment for ME throughout the period from 2002 to today and many articles and research papers have given some support to the use of this therapy despite the costs involved in training staff and monitoring the individual's progress. These therapies propose that patients should be encouraged to

---

[21] *BMJ* 2013;347:f5731

change their illness beliefs and gradually increase their activities. The author recognised the shortcomings of this approach in a NICE judicial review in 2007:

> It is also misleading to refer to CBT & GET as 'treatments' of choice'. They cannot properly be described as treatments, since, as NICE admits, they do not address the core pathology of ME. Neither is there effective choice given that many patients will be denied much of the knowledge they need to make informed decisions and there is little alternative to CBT and GET on offer in the NHS. CBT/GET have also been rejected by some ME patient charities in the UK. The NICE Guidelines give the false impression, to doctors, politicians, and the MRC, that effective treatments are available for ME patients. NICE would do better honestly to admit that their core therapy recommendations are not properly evidence-based, and to use this admission as the starting point for an adequately funded search for a cure. We should not forget that ME patients have a legitimate right to aspire to a cure. [22]

The PACE Trial study by a consortium of UK research units in 2011 erupted into controversy and its results continue to be challenged. Dr David Tuller of University of California, Berkeley questioned the methodology and findings of the study[23] claiming that the psychosocial view of ME has not benefited from the $8 million investment and has set the interest in the search for a cure backwards. The *640* Trial participants were chosen to undergo a series of 4 therapeutic treatments and monitored under 2 categories: Fatigue and Physical function. The results were widely criticised for suggesting considerable improvements were gained

---

[22] Gibson I. Witness statement in support of the Judicial Review case of the NICE "CFS/ME" Guideline (CG53) online brought by ME patients: Re: Douglas Fraser & Kevin Short v NICE Case Number: CO/10408/2007. Exclusion code: 9.

[23] Trial by Error: The Troubling Case of the PACE Chronic Fatigue Syndrome Study. www.virology.ws/2015/10/21/trial-by-error-i

from the treatments applied: Adaptive Pacing, Cognitive Behavioural Therapy, Graded Exercise Therapy or stand along Specialist Medical Care. The treatments offered different ways for patients to deal with and improve the symptoms of CFS/ME and its effects on disability. The results of the PACE Trial were published in The Lancet in 2011 and further results in subsequent papers. The controversial results indicate that the attitudes and behaviour of those suffering from ME have a role to play in the long-term continuation of their debilitating condition.

> This 'behavioural' explanation has long been the source of voracious criticism and questioning of the PACE Trial protocols, evaluations and secrecy surrounding patients' medical profiles. Several Freedom of Information requests were made to Queen Mary College London (QMUL) about the details of the Trial since The Lancet article was published in 2011. All were initially refused and QMUL were rumoured to have spent over £200k in legal fees in attempts to avoid the data being released. The original protocol under which the trial was initially funded was changed during the course of the trial and so QMUL claimed that the information requested was based on a changed protocol for the Trial and not available following the changes. ME charities and advocates continued to pursue their requests through the UK legislative process and eventually some of the data was released [24]

Initial analysis and comparison of the released data then showed a huge discrepancy between the claimed improvements from the official trial and the results using the original published protocol. The difference was in fact threefold – rendering the trial statistically insignificant and of no value in treating ME.

---

[24]

http://www.informationtribunal.gov.uk/DBFiles/Decision/i1854/Queen%20Mary%20University%20of%20London%20EA-2015-0269%20(12-8-16).PDF

Cognitive Behavioral Therapy (CBT) is about examining how thoughts, behavior and CFS/ME symptoms interact with each other. Between therapy sessions, participants in this treatment group are encouraged to try out new ways of coping with their illness. CBT has been recommended to doctors treating ME patients in the UK for several years The NHS quotes both terms ME and CFS for the illness depending on the specificity of symptoms, but also introduces the new name *Systemic Exertion Intolerance Disease* (SEID) – a term suggested in a 2015 report by the US Institute of Medicine, which implies that the condition affects many systems in the body (systemic); the word "disease" highlights the serious nature of the condition in some people.

Definitions and Prevalence

Research is being undertaken in Bristol and elsewhere in the UK to identify the number of cases of ME with different definitions. Two studies led by a University of Bristol-led research team were awarded a grant of £1.2 million by the Department for Health in 2013. The first project for £864,000 is a 5-year study entitled 'Investigating the treatment of paediatric chronic fatigue syndrome or myalgic encephalomyelitis' with a multi-centre trial on children with ME, their treatment and recovery rates, including the success of Graded Exercise Therapy as one of the treatments currently recommended by the NHS.

The other Bristol led study funded with £32,861 over 3-years is entitled 'CFS in the NHS: diagnosis of Chronic Fatigue Syndrome in primary care and outcomes after treatment by specialist services'. One member of the research team is Dr Simon Collin who says "Approximately 9,000 adults are assessed annually by NHS specialist CFS/ME services in England, of whom approximately 80 per cent are diagnosed with CFS/ME.

Assessment rates vary six-fold across England with specialist services using a range of treatments with little or no standardisation across the NHS. The extent to which patients recover from their illness and are able to return to normal activity levels is unknown" [25] although a 2012 study led by Dr David Bell from New York, USA, suggested that over time many individuals will not maintain a CFS diagnosis but they will not return to their premorbid level of functioning.

This is complemented by studies on prognosis of the illness and its development as a chronic condition in contrast to the levels of impairment experienced in other well-known conditions.

There is a great deal of unease – partly due to the amount of funding that has been awarded for these studies and also because many view these studies as conflating chronic fatigue, chronic fatigue syndrome and ME, thus influencing prevalence figures for ME incorrectly.

The NHS and ME

It appears that the majority of patients presenting with symptoms of ME in the UK are still referred to psychotherapists for treatment. GPs have been given little or no training in alternative biomedical interventions and so the answers are sought in cognitive behavioral therapy (CBT) and lifestyle regimes. The official description of ME by the NHS states:

It is estimated around 250,000 people in the UK have CFS. Anyone can get the condition, although it's more common in women than men. It usually develops when people are in their early 20s to mid-40s. Children can also be affected, usually between the ages of 13 and 15"

---

[25] www.bris.ac.uk/news/2013/9741.html, 2015

and the treatment recommended:

"cognitive behavioural therapy (CBT); a structured exercise programme *called* graded exercise therapy (GET); medication to control pain, nausea and sleeping problems. [26]

The question arises as to how the number of 250,000 has been calculated? If General Practitioners do reach the correct diagnosis of ME, where is this recorded?

To our knowledge there is no official calculation, but perhaps the Minister of Health can correct us on this?

Like cancer treatment, early diagnosis with rest can help as can self-treatment. One case that demonstrates this pathway is that of Ida, a Norwegian student who fell ill with ME during a field trip to Uganda in 2002. Back in the UK she received an early diagnosis of ME from an informed doctor and, at this time of poor knowledge about the disease, scant research and only psychological treatment, she built her own programme of recovery over several years with rest, diet and self-pacing to rebuild her health.

This particular case illustrates how an early diagnosis can allow a patient to self-help towards recovery or at least stabilising their condition, armed with the knowledge available in books and on the Internet. Many others in our experience are unable to get the correct diagnosis. This is still too often because the medical approach invites denial that ME exists. We include here the story of one person's pathway over 10 years of suffering from ME in both the UK and Norway.

---

[26] www.nhs.uk/conditions/chronic-fatigue-syndrome, 2015

Case Study: Ida

When I first met Ida she was a dynamic, enthusiastic student of international development and natural resources who came from Norway to study for a BSc at a university in the UK. Always cheerful and enthusiastic, she was well liked by staff and students. Ida went to Uganda for a period of research on her undergraduate programme and fell ill with a debilitating disease called Bilharzias, also known as Schistosomiasis. This infection comes from parasites living in fresh water rivers and lakes in subtropical or tropical zones. Symptoms often develop within a few weeks and include flu-like symptoms, fever and aching muscle. If treatment is not given, or is unsuccessful, the disease can lead to long-term problems such as stomach pains and cramps and paralysis of the legs. However, Ida returned to the UK several weeks later.

> It was whilst I was doing my research I was ill, for a week, I think, it may have been longer than a week and I was really low and I was examined at a clinic and they couldn't really find anything wrong with me, I can't even remember if I had any medication or if I just had to rest and just pick myself up again. This was in Uganda while doing my research. I was just totally drained. It was probably midway through my research - it was for 3 months - and at some point I was really not feeling well but I don't think they figured out what it was. Yes, I had to get going again to continue with my research and I think I was OK. But coming back to England when I was still feeling low I was checked for all sorts of diseases and they found bilharzias in my blood and so I was treated for that. It's easy treatment, you just take some pills and you're fine. I had nothing diagnosed apart from bilharzias. I contracted that from swimming in a lake near Kabala in South West Uganda.
>
> I became increasingly tired after completing my dissertation

and it must have been after I handed in my dissertation, I went on a 2 week trip back to Uganda as a research facilitator at a workshop organized by X and Y about field techniques for assessing soil degradation. I was the assistant facilitator for that workshop and I was just really, really tired and completing my degree became increasingly difficult, but I managed to complete my degree.......

The process of excluding other diseases began in 2001 with my doctor. The diagnosis took several months I think because as various tests had to be done in order to exclude other illnesses and there was a doctor at the University Health Centre whose working hypothesis was that it was ME but he had to exclude everything else. So once everything else was excluded he concluded that yes, it was ME. I had blood tests and we talked a lot as well..... We talked a lot about my childhood and my upbringing. I think I kind of paused and reflected on a whole lot of issues and I think everything just.... it was a combination of things, but resting obviously didn't make matters any better so no matter how much I rested, how much I exercised, I couldn't really pick myself up again like I would normally have done.

At this point Ida decided to return to her parents' home in Norway where she was cared for by both her parents and her partner. All were supportive in their own ways. The focus of the health care she received in Norway between 2002-11 was based on the assumption that she had psychological problems rather than ME.

In 2002 I moved back to Norway and I don't think I came across any doctors in Norway who had any experience with ME and the treatment but the doctor I was seeing had heard that anti-depressants could be beneficial in treating ME. So I was prescribed anti-depressants. I don't think there was any treatment, there was nothing. I did some research on my own and there was an ME association in my town and I read a lot about ME...... The symptoms made sense. I was always really thirsty and very light sensitive and it took a lot of energy just thinking about getting dressed and once I had gotten dressed I was totally, totally drained. It was like OK, right, I need to sit down and watch TV. I watched a lot of TV, because that relaxed me. I could just sit and observe. So I was never bed ridden for days and days and days, but I couldn't really function.

From the literature I read I knew it was not psychological, that it was neurological but it's intertwined with your psychology – how your mental health is affected by your illness. So I don't think I was under the impression that the cause was an illness in my head, it was not like a psychological disease, but my conclusion was that I was under physical and emotional stress over the years that had culminated in this Chronic Fatigue Syndrome and I heard all sorts of things about vaccinations being the cause and I guess I never put any energy into researching it and going down that road to figure out if any of my vaccinations caused ME.

I read literature and knew how to treat the ME through eating food that wasn't processed and sort of giving your body clean food so that it wouldn't struggle with additives and other chemicals. So organic and stone age, paleo diet. My parents didn't want to recognize that I suffered mentally, for a variety of reasons...... it took a while for them to realize that I was really ill. So if I walked downstairs and had to go back up again for some reason, I felt I couldn't, I had to rest. I was always expected to be the one I was before I was ill, to run errands, do people favours, to do this and do that. I remember being absolutely incapable of doing anything. Just existing. My parents and brothers and friends didn't understand, they hadn't heard of ME.

I didn't think there was any treatment. There were some pills I used to dilute in water and I had read that it was beneficial for people with ME to strengthen the immune system, increase energy levels. I think it was an alternative health professional, through a natural food store….. I can't remember the name. I used to take a lot of dietary supplements. I think I saw an ad in the paper about the ME association so I went to a few meetings but by that time I had read a lot of books, a lot of literature about it. I don't think I felt that it was of benefit for me to attend the meetings because I had already found my way to deal with it. So I wasn't an active part of that group.

If I told people I had ME they said "What's that?" they hadn't heard of it. I would use the WHO description because in 2002 it was a recognized disease. I don't think people questioned it. Once they got the explanation no one understood it and no-one understands it, but they accepted that, OK, yes, she has these symptoms and it is ME and this is a mysterious illness……. From what I had understood people who got ME were very driven and take on a lot of responsibility and are seen as having a huge capacity for work, they seem to be more susceptible to ME. Yes, resourceful people are just suddenly knocked flat out with ME. I read about this in published articles, books been written, research being done and case studies, so it wasn't like a slow disease. So you would be going full steam ahead and then, whoosh, you would be stopped dead in your tracks…… I found my own way to deal with it. I was back on my feet. It took quite some years before I was fully functioning again, maybe until 2005-6 maybe in 2007-8, physically yes. I was still taking the anti-depressants till 2011.

By 2004 Ida felt well enough to return to the UK and embark

on an MRes course for one year that normally leads to three years of study for a PhD. When I saw Ida again in late 2004 I could see that she was not fully recovered. She seemed a shadow of her former self and bit by bit she fell back into a state of constant fatigue. In 2005, after just 9 months, Ida had to give up her studies and returned to Norway.

On her return to Norway in 2005 Ida was back to zero energy levels and facing an uncertain future. As a strong willed character she decided that, with the lack of professional help, she would have to find her own way back to health. She was also fortunate in having the support of her family and her partner during this time.

Firstly, I had to recognize that this was real, not an illness that I could snap out of. I had to work my way out of it. My energy level went to zero. I remember hitting rock bottom was when I was living with my boyfriend and his son, where my parents were …. and I remember being in the bath and so exhausted that I just wanted to sink beneath the water. Ok it's not the solution I want. But just the thought of getting up, drying myself off, putting my clothes on…. Just that effort, I can't do it. I can't do it.

So how did Ida deal with this state of utter fatigue?

I just need to be on my own and have no other responsibilities but to look after me. I spent a lot of time preparing food for myself. I was avoiding processed food. I read a book called 'Tired of Being Tired'[27] it was about Chronic Fatigue Syndrome I think, a very good book, I think that was the book that helped me the most. I had a lot of books about ME but that book had a lot of recipes and it explained a lot of stuff

---

[27] Hanley, Jesse L. and Deville, Nancy (2002) Tired of Being Tired: Rescue, Repair, Rejuvenate

about my body that was absolutely drained and I had to replenish.

It was kind of like having the flu non-stop, not really headaches. I was sensitive to light. I couldn't be in a room full of people, that would totally exhaust me and I could focus on a one to one basis with people. I remember driving a car and I would do exactly the opposite of what you were supposed to do. I start to drive at the red light and stop at the green. My brain didn't function. I couldn't trust myself to make the right decisions driving in traffic and I couldn't drive at night because at night when you have the sharp headlights coming towards you, it was just too much. It was a long road to recovery. …. I don't think I'm as strong as I was before ME, but of course age is a factor.

Our thanks go to Ida (not her real name) for sharing her story with us for this book.

Part 2 - Current and future research
The Struggle Continues

The causes of ME are, of course, still unknown and so this division of views between those who advocate 'behavioural' explanations and others who support a physical explanation persists. There are others who believe we should not be approaching the problem by assuming that there are various symptoms representing different conditions. As we discovered, certain questions should be framed in terms of research funding, recognising that we should be supporting good research without the assumption that we have an answer. We discuss in Chapter 3 how this bilateral debate has been politically manipulated and in Chapter 4 perhaps the underlying reason why ME has been so severely affected by policy-based evidence making.

Research into the known symptoms has lent force to a plethora of potential directions (and businesses), e.g. drugs, homeopathy, cognitive therapies, acupuncture, dietary treatment etc. The establishment favoured treatments are graded exercise therapy (GET) and cognitive behavioural therapy (CBT).

The Medical Research Council's Summary Report on CFS/ME published in 2003 urged research to move on with clinical trials for effective treatment before the cause and development of ME/CFS had been fully understood. This had also been the case with diabetes, where development of treatment preceded knowledge of the cause and development of the disease. The MRC officially state that they encourage collaboration in research from patients, carers and health professionals yet some doubt their intent based on their actions to date. Patients and support groups helping to set the agenda enrich a research strategy and scientists can gain access to perspectives on the patients that help frame research questions.

Oxford University, King's College London, Queen Mary University London, University of Bristol and Newcastle University feature in a network where allocation of grants followed. This reflects the predominance of university research money being given to the 'Golden Triangle' of London, Oxford and Cambridge in the UK. Other universities get little look in and often exist on charitable support that ignites new pathways of research. You have to publish results and that becomes difficult in a world populated by an 'elite' who think they know what the answer is likely to be and control the allocation of financial resources, awards and personal plaudits for chosen scientists. Woe betides the individual who steps outside the box in research work or goes to the press to complain of any of these factors. This was a feature in the events surrounding the Incline outbreak of ME in the USA.

Without understanding the underlying mechanisms in a disease any development of a therapeutic treatment will stall without well-researched markers of the disease. It is difficult to set up trials with complete blinding of samples and treatments, since it can be like comparing oranges with apples. So watertight definitions are needed for each patient to allow proper monitoring with any therapy. We have become familiar with genetic environmental and internal factors having an association with a condition but in ME there has been little discussion or research into gene mutations, identical and non-identical twins (they do exist in ME) and also initial viral infections seem to play a role. So some researchers are now talking of 'switching' of a regulatory feedback position to some abnormal state initially set up by a series of unpredictable events. Scientists are now looking at the remission of ME and the causes of this. Areas of research include changes in leucocyte[28] gene expression, autonomic nerve cell dysfunction, herpes virus immune response and cytokine levels some of which may occur at high levels in early stages of the illness. A large number of causative factors – viral infection, immune activation, exposure to toxins, chemicals and pesticides, low intensity radiation and electromagnetic fields – have been suggested as aetiological factors (multifactorial disease). Altered gene expression profiles in ME patient populations have been reported. Pathways of disease development involve metabolic dysregulation as a chronic pathological state. Mitochondrial dysfunction also has been proposed for ME. Similarity to the pathways observed in ageing with mitochondrial[29] and cellular enzyme concentration and/or decrease in activity could explain the similarity with ageing processes.

---

[28] Leucocyte = white blood cells in the immune system.
[29] Mitochondria = Mitochondria are found in every cell of the human body except red blood cells, and convert the energy of food molecules into the biochemical reaction that powers most cell functions.

There are, apparently, some ongoing physiological disturbances involving the immune system in our bodies, the central nervous system and even several pathways of interaction may be involved. What a primary event and a secondary event are remains mysterious and recent work in mitochondrial dysfunction may be a secondary event. So how does the brain respond to autoimmune[30] effects in the body or to infection, or even to variations in the gut microbiome[31]? Brain abnormalities may involve the microglia[32] associated with persistent pain and this could be caused by a virus for example, and lead to effects in the autonomic pathways. Others have related the symptoms to research, signalling pathways being rendered abnormal. Whilst this is a confusing picture, it might all emanate from one particular piece of the physiological chain. The research into these areas of immune cell reaction in ME could provide key information and eradicate the still prevailing ideology of 'middle class shirkers'. The gun has been fired and the scientists are running. However, they need real encouragement and support.

In the rest of this chapter we will discuss some of the research particularly involving B cell depletion as part of immune disorder. Unravelling secondary effects is possible in gene expression levels but leaves the jury out on one initial cause of these events. The effects of certain treatments e.g. with antidepressants, has not led to an association with neuro-transmissions. These approaches could be said to be peripheral but interesting enough to require more research. There are many new leads in the areas and more international scientific cooperation is needed. How to develop political support for the efforts are addressed in our next chapter.

---

[30] Autoimmune = reaction of an individual to their own cells.
[31] Microbiome = the *human microbiome* is composed of the microbes, as well as their genes and genomes, that live in and on the *human* body.
[32] Microglia = a cell found in the brain and spinal cord which acts as the first and main form of active immune defence in the central nervous system.

The first priority according to Professor Jonathan Edwards (University College London) is to form links between epidemiologists, clinical academics and laboratory researchers. Epidemiological facts played an important role in rheumatoid arthritis and population studies for genetic understanding of other diseases. As with recent advances in cancer research, understanding immunological processes can play a huge role in developing new treatments. For example, natural killer cells, cytokine changes and immune responses to viruses like EBV (Epstein-Barr Virus) need research. Auto-antibodies for neural chemicals or cellular receptors is a fascinating area of study. As Edwards and his collaborators found out, following the October 2015 European ME Research Group Meeting, the door is now open in these and other areas. He points out in his joint paper that 'prognosis for ME is poor and the impact of current care limited'. Strategically he says, as a successful researcher in other fields of medicine 'comparable problems have been familiar in research into other disabling conditions in the past and many cases have been alleviated by major progress in recent years. '

Some of this work is underway in Australia, the UK, Sweden, Norway, Germany and in the USA. Let us look specifically, however, at cytokines. The general hypothesis is that ME can result in overwhelming fatigue and cognitive difficulties. It was classified by the World Health Organisation in 1969 as a neurological category. We know that research should focus on cytokines entering the brain. Cytokines are molecules that help cells communicate with each other in response to inflammation, infection or trauma. They are part of the immune system and are associated with ME. More intense research is needed on the role of cytokines when signs of neuro-inflammation are present. Natural killer (NK) cells change functionality, a common feature associated with herpes virus infection (from the 6th Invest in ME Research Biomedical Research Colloquium in 2016) and other viral infections. Research in immune system activation using the measurement of cytokine in blood leads scientists to observe that this can cause patients to suffer from flu-like symptoms commonly found with ME. There have been several suggestions that there are changes in the immune system of those suffering from ME but so far there has been no agreement about the type and extent of these changes and how they affect the development of the disease.

The effect on the gut microbiota is also under investigation. The balance between our gut microbiota and our immune system is important for inflammatory and autoimmune disease patterns. Maybe this leads the ME patients to problems in the bowel and a so-called leaky gut barrier. The products from the gut bacteria and viruses may affect our immune cells and hence cause inflammation on the pathway to the brain. This exciting new work is occurring in Norwich and Oxford in the UK and Cornell and Columbia universities in the USA. As Professor Tom Wileman pointed out in the IIMEC11 conference in London 2016, viruses and bacteria may act in complex ways to affect the balance of the organisms in our gut and affect various behavioural and biological pathways.

It is important to add that infections in our gut can cause anxiety, depression and cognitive changes. In 2003 the MRC Research Advisory Group for CFS/ME concluded that:

Psychological factors, including personality, coping mechanisms and social support, play a role in the manifestations of all illnesses, however well-established their physical causes. A problem with CFS/ME is that it is not clear at what point in the illness psychological factors may well play a part. [33]

---

[33] New Research Directions for CFS/ME. (2003) Medical Research Council

Prominent Research into ME

Much of the biological research into ME in the UK has been funded by charities. Invest in ME Research is currently funding research in the UK on a gut microbiome project at UEA/IFR (the University of East Anglia and Institute for Food Research). PhD students are being recruited to continue research. Invest in ME Research is supporting research into the link between autoimmunity and ME. The approach addresses the possible link between neuro-inflammation and systemic infections of the body. Our gastrointestinal tracts contain millions of bacteria and viruses that can affect intestinal barrier function and host defences against microbial changes that can lead to chronic inflammation. Any research into ME can be addressed by examining ME and non-ME patients.

Invest in ME Research funded research on B cells has just been published in Clinical & Experimental Immunology and this work continues under the leadership of Dr Jo Cambridge, Professorial Research Associate at UCL. It is being done in collaboration with researchers in Bergen, Norway where B cell depletion therapy has been trialled and continues to be trialled as a treatment for ME patients. In addition, Invest in ME Research initiated and arranged for the European ME Research Group (EMERG) - a group of European researchers collaborating and sharing knowledge, meeting in London at the Invest in ME Research conference in 2016. Also organized by Invest in ME Research are the 7th Biomedical Research into ME Colloquium and the 12th International ME in June 2017 [34] (see Annex 1).

One significant move is that several European countries and the USA have established bio-banks of biological material to be available for future research and which can be shared across nations. Peterson and his colleagues at Simmaron in Nevada are

---

[34] http://www.investinme.eu

developing new translational science approaches for ME in their large research unit. The unit has a repository of over 1,000 patient biological samples and these records form a rich resource for research as do the samples being collected and stored by Drs Mella and Fluge at Haukeland University Hospital in Bergen, Norway, and elsewhere. In other centres in the States neuro-immunological work and viral effects on the process are actively under scrutiny by Chia, Knox and Montoya.

At Columbia University's Mailman School of Public Health, Mady Hornig and Ian Lipkin have identified distinct immune changes in patients diagnosed with ME. Using blood samples they have found specific biomarkers in patients up to 3 years with the disease. Therefore, diagnosis could be made much earlier if the results hold up. Hornig is also making interesting observations on cytokines at different stages in the development of ME. In particular, however, biomarkers for ME at whatever stage would herald a big breakthrough in identification and classification of ME.

Another welcome initiative in the research associated with ME has recently come from the USA. The National Institute of Health has determined to advance research on ME a disease for which an accurate diagnosis and effective treatment has remained elusive. They are discussing the details of a research protocol to study individuals and have set up a working group including the National Institute of Neurological Disorders and Stroke to ensure the multi-institute research efforts. The NIH director, Francis Collins, a distinguished scientist has high hopes of finding a cause and new preventions and treatment can be initiated. A recent Institute of Medicine report in the USA under President Obama's direction has set a new diagnostic criteria and a new name – Systemic Exertion Intolerance Disease (SEID). We interviewed one of those involved in this report in the USA, Dr Dan Peterson, who advised us to "wait and see if the Institute of Medicine document leads to financial support and action. Obama may want to go with a flourish". However, the NIH representative at the Invest in ME Research London conference in 2016 heralded the new money for research into ME without prejudice. Dr Whittemore contributed to the debates to accentuate how she was committed to the NIH programme of 6 million dollars (Lyme disease gets 20 million dollars) for research. She encouraged European scientists to consider applying for grants.

Ampligen

There is at the moment no effective treatment or cure. As Dan Peterson, a founding member of Simmaron Research, said to the author, Ian Gibson, at a conference in 2015 - "we have various treatments that are popular here or there and I treat many patients using Ampligen" - whilst others exercise or get treatment such as cognitive behavioural therapy.

The drug Ampligen is produced by a Philadelphia based company called Hemispherx Biopharma Inc and is described by the company as an experimental nucleic acid which is "being developed for the potential treatment of globally important viral diseases and disorders of the immune system including Human Papillomavirus (HPV), Human Immune Deficiency Virus (HIV), Chronic Fatigue Syndrome (CFS), Hepatitis and influenza."[35] The drug has also been used on mice during 2015 in laboratory experiments for treating Ebola. The company claims that more than 40,000 doses at over 20 U.S. clinical trial sites have been delivered by Ampligen®. Over 500 patients were given Ampligen intravenously and results show that 80% of patients claim an

---

[35] www.hemispherx.net 2015

improvement and 50% a significant improvement (Hunter-Hopkins Centre). The treatment is currently only permitted in trials under conditional permits issued by the Federal Drug Agency (FDA).

At the time of writing Ampligen is currently listed as an experimental drug although Hemispherx claim that large amounts of money have been spent on research and trials to meet FDA's requirements for approval. Patients have been waiting for over 20 years for a drug to alleviate the main symptoms of ME and so the lack of FDA approval has been a source of great frustration, not just in the USA, but also throughout the world. Patients we spoke to in Sweden said that Ampligen was not currently available in Scandinavia but if it became available anywhere else in Europe they were willing to travel at their own expense in order to purchase the drug.

As it turns out Hemispherx Biopharma [36] announced in July that rintatolimod (Ampligen) was being made available for CFS patients, under early access regulations in the EU. Then in August the company announced that it has received approval of its New Drug Application from Administracion Nacional de Medicamentos, Alimentos y Tecnologia Medica (ANMAT) for commercial sale of rintatolimod in the Argentine Republic for the treatment of severe myalgic encephalomyelitis/chronic fatigue syndrome (ME/CFS). Rintatolimod would therefore become the first drug to receive approval of this kind anywhere in the world.

Rituximab

In Norway, Fluge and Mella (2011) have shown that the depletion of B-lymphocyte cells in patients suffering with ME can lead to

---

[36] http://www.nasdaq.com/press-release/hemispherx-biopharma-to-present-at-the-18th-annual-rodman--renshaw-global-investment-conference-20160906-00553#/ixzz4JUjfI1TR

dramatic changes in self-reported fatigue scores. These cells depleting in number mean fewer antibodies, clogs in blood vessel permeation and the movement of other cells (lymphocytes) to sites of injury. The Norwegian collaboration is examining the effects of the drug rituximab on the B cell populations of people with ME. Øystein Fluge and Olav Mella of the Haukeland University Hospital in Bergen published a report in 2011 suggesting that the symptoms of ME could be treated positively with the drug rituximab (Fluge et al, PLoS ONE 2011). However, they are careful in their claims of remission and we await the results when the drug has gone through all clinical trials currently underway. Rituximab is a drug commonly used in certain cancer treatments and autoimmune disorders. The report and its clinical findings showed that on the Rituximab Trial 67% of patients on rituximab had lasting improvements in self-reported fatigue compared to only 13% on the placebo. These findings immediately drew the attention of scientists, ME charities and patients. Extensive media coverage followed– though it was barely mentioned in the UK media, unlike the attention freely and immediately given to research that attempts to highlight the benefits of CBT and GET. A second trial produced similar results and reported on the continued use of the drug on patients from the first trial: "Eleven of the 18 responders were still in remission three years after beginning the treatment, and some have now had no symptoms for five years...Suddenly, their limbs started to work again and their hands were no longer cold or sweaty." [37]

More clinical trials are being planned, including one in the UK. This research will receive support from the Invest in ME Research Biomedical Research Programme and hopefully be advanced with public funding eventually. Another possible source of funding is

---

[37] B-Lymphocyte depletion in myalgic encephalopathy/chronic fatigue syndrome. An open-label phase II study with rituximab maintenance treatment. Fluge Ø, et al. PLoS One, 2015 Jul 1; 10(7): e0129898.

expected from collaborative meetings with various European countries and applications for funding are planned to the European Parliament from its Health budget. Collaboration is underway between Drs Fluge and Mella at the Haukeland University Hospital in Bergen, Norway and with Dr Jo Cambridge and her team at University College London and also planned with colleagues at the Norwich Research Park and University of East Anglia. There are two main types of lymphocytes in the human body. One is B-lymphocytes (B cells) and the other is T-lymphocytes (T cells). The latter augment or suppress immune responses and attack bacteria. B cells produce immunoglobulins which bind to and help kill bacteria and viruses. These cells are active in destroying tumours. Along with her student Fane Mensah, Jo Cambridge is studying the B cell subsets as the disease develops and beginning to see some patterns of cell development. It is still early days yet.

These studies are being complemented by the work in Berlin with auto-antibodies involving neuro transmitter receptors and their presence after rituximab treatment. It remains to be seen if there is a tie up with specific receptors. The central thesis here is to identify B cell populations and how they are affected by infections with e.g. the Epstein-Barr virus. B cells are key to antibody production, an important feature of attacking, for example, bacteria. They interact with T cells in antibody formation through the production of cytokines. The latter either rise or fall in ME, as also shown by Mady Hornig. The variation between individuals in e.g. producing numbers of B cells needs a clearer understanding. Finally, the work of Eleanor Riley in the UK in the search for biomarkers concentrates on changes in immune cells (NK and T cells) after infection.

At Newcastle University, with the support of the MRC, Professor Newton and Dr Wan Ng are exploring in depth autonomic dysfunction and its association with neuro-cognitive impairments. They are also looking at gene expression in blood to enable them to profile biological fingerprints for fatigue. In California Andreas Kogelnik is developing information on ME patients and any genetic influences. This follows up the work by Jonathan Kerr in the UK. In Australia at Griffiths University, Sonya Marshall-Gradisnik and Don Staines are taking a molecular biological approach, to find the signature of autoimmune responses through molecules allied with genetic characteristics and are identifying targets for potential medical interventions. They are claiming interesting results from DNA changes as well as NK cells in patients.

Jonas Bergquist from Sweden has looked at many of the proteins at different stages in the development of ME and is encouraged by some of the changes he sees. Luis Nacul in London believes that ME should not be compared with CFS as the former has more symptoms.

Amolak Bansal, also in the UK, has tried to research the process of diagnosis in ME. He has a scoring system[38] to identify an ME population. He is beginning to see significant differences between the symptoms of patients. He has been less successful so far in identifying trigger infections and he is looking at effects of vaccination. He seems intent on looking at patients through various periods of relapse and remission. At the recent Invest in ME Research BRMEC6 Research Colloquium in 2016 he pointed out how any stress could set up a chain of biochemical changes.

To sum up, some of the more challenging research is now entering interesting areas. We should also mention:

(a) Neil Harrison in the UK who is looking at inflammation following depression, work which may have a relevance for ME.

---

[38] https://bmcfampract.biomedcentral.com/articles/10.1186/s12875-016-0493-0

(b) John Chia in the USA who has some exciting observations on enteroviruses and is accumulating much new evidence on how they present in the human body.

(c) Carmen Scheibenbogen in Germany is interested in B cell sub-populations which attract the Epstein-Barr virus (EBV). The presence of this virus can be tracked by viral proteins at different stages of B cell growth.

Another interesting approach is that again demonstrated through Norwegian research. It is often asked if an illness is genetic – runs in families – and in the last few years' research on twins, identical or fraternal and family studies have been carried out on cancers and many other illnesses. Little has been done with ME, probably because definitions vary across borders. However, in the Department of Oncology at Haukeland University Hospital in Oslo, preliminary work shows there is an increased risk in 1st degree relatives and even 2nd degree. The scientists are looking at DNA sequences to see if they can identify the gene. Using new molecular biological techniques applied with other illnesses there is the prospect of identifying genes that play a major role in the development of ME. At the same time, discussions are underway in Norwich, UK to set up studies in twins to see if ME correlates with genetic identity.

Molecular techniques have not received the support necessary to look at questions of genetic causes but new supporters of the techniques are emerging from the USA as well as Norway. Mitochondrial genomes are being investigated at Cornell University in the States and interesting DNA variants are turning up in association with inflammations of the brain and gastro-intestinal symptoms.

Recently, in London at the Invest in ME Research IIMEC11 conference, Maureen Hanson from the USA, described her work on mitochondria from patients and the relevance of biochemical drugs that she has recorded. Professor Elisa Oltra from the Catholic University in Valencia, Spain described her research looking for molecular biomarkers in patients and again has encouraging studies underway with enzymes and micro-RNA molecules. There must surely be some progress in the biomarker research in the next year or so given the activity. Ron Davis from Stanford University in the USA described his Big Data approach and his talk was well received. No doubt with its philosophy and support from computer technologies, it will help the focus on the likely areas of research to give results. His approach mirrors the research interactions between physicists, chemists, mathematicians, computer technologists etc. across the piste.

Finally, several other groups in the USA and the UK are looking at ME via brain imaging processes at patients with ME and those without it, whether at a later stage in the development of ME or in an early phase. This makes for an exciting piece of research. There have so far been many inconsistent measurements of the detailed responses of patients in their immune system e.g. cytokine measurement in blood samples and different laboratory technologies are often one answer. Much more research needs to be done in those areas outlined above. We should always bear in mind there may be different individual responses to similar onslaughts of infections. What is clear is that these biochemical and physiological observations may be significant explanations of the illness and further research will be encouraged.

Recently this review of autoimmune diseases was highlighted in a Science magazine article 'Fighting autoimmunity with immune cells – A way forward':

Autoimmune diseases share a grim similarity with cancer. People's own cells become their enemies. But a study published online in Science reveals a happier parallel, suggesting that a therapy designed to harness the immune system to attack cancer cells may also cull the turncoat immune cells behind certain autoimmune diseases. The approach relies on chimeric antigen receptor T cells, or CAR T cells: immune cells genetically modified to home in on a desired target on cancer cells or – in this case – on rogue B cells, another immune cell type. The new study only gauged the CAR T cells' capabilities in the lab dish and in mouse models of pemphigus vulgaris, an autoimmune condition in which B cells secrete antibodies that attack a protein in skin and mucous membrane. But some scientists are already calling the approach, which specifically targets the errant B cells, a breakthrough. [39]

To conclude this pot-pourri of current research, it was Professor Ron Davis who said in London at the IIMEC11 conference that 'if you are looking for fish you have to go fishing'. It is difficult, if not impossible, to say at this stage what are more likely to be the prolific areas. However, the increase in the number of laboratories and countries entering the research fray are encouraging. Since we are witnessing the gradual build up in biomedical research in ME we have talked to students early in careers who may or may not teach or even research with ME in medical faculties. This should be encouraged as much as possible.

Student Interviews

One difficulty in engaging the research aspirations of medical students in ME is the lack of information at undergraduate level in both the UK and Europe. Two recently qualified medical students from the Netherlands (although trained in the UK) told us there was barely a mention of ME in their medical training and they remained unclear on how to define ME, let alone how to treat it.

We interviewed two of the earlier students who were carrying out

---

[39] Leslie, Mitch 'Fighting autoimmunity with immune cells' *Science*, 14: 1 July, 2016

research into ME in Norwich, funded by Invest in ME Research. They had been convinced of its value and interest following discussions with Professor Wileman. They had received no lecture material mentioning ME in their medical training. As pioneers they had struggled to get ME blood samples due to the inaccessibility of patients in the Norfolk area. Each time they needed to access samples meant a 150 mile round trip. One student had made 60 such trips. Getting the ethical permission to approach the patients was helped by the local consultant, but red tape delayed the whole process of getting the patients and then their permission. It was difficult, they said, but they felt the research was interesting i.e. microbiome studies of the gut. They had had to face teasing and ridicule from fellow peer group students who said 'ME wasn't real'! At the 2016 BRMEC6 Colloquium a consultant related that of his colleagues in the hospital only 2 out of 50 believed ME was real.

'It shows you what we are up against' he said.

The importance of a laboratory being in close contact with patients in a very local hospital was paramount for their research. Efforts are being made to enable this to be a feature of the Centre of Excellence for ME in Norwich.

One of them was now a junior doctor and the other was unsure of the best future career to pursue. There were worries about the long term future of jobs in sciences and medicine as they had witnessed good work being withdrawn from funding streams.

At a conference called 'De Osynliga' (The Invisible Ones) organised by European ME Alliance Sweden member RME (National Association for ME Patients) in Stockholm, October 2015, we met two young women who are identical twins. One twin has chronic ME, the other was concerned that she was experiencing the first symptoms. Research into the implications of

ME affecting identical twins needs further exploration and could reveal genetic information related to the pathology of the illness.

Chapter 3 - How the Story Unfolds

Definitions

What is a disease?

'A disorder of structure or function in a human, animal, or plant, especially one that produces specific signs or symptoms or that affects a specific location and is not simply a direct result of physical injury.'

What is a virus?

'An infective agent that typically consists of a nucleic acid molecule in a protein coat, is too small to be seen by light microscopy, and is able to multiply only within the living cells of a host.'

(Oxford English Dictionary)

Whenever a previously unknown disease or virus appears there is conjecture and fear. The media, newspapers, TV and radio, and these days social media, play a large part in forming initial understandings of both cause and possible treatments. The outbreak of HIV/AIDS, SARS, Ebola, West Nile virus, Zika and frequent flu epidemics are examples of sensational media coverage often leading to misconceptions and social stigmatisation both locally and globally. The story of HIV/AIDS is well known and demonstrates how the first reactions, based on incomplete factual, scientific knowledge, led to false interpretations and the personification of victims as immoral by those with extreme religious views who believed it was divine retribution for the practice of homosexuality. The impact on society is huge – sexual and racial discrimination, shunning of individuals, creating metaphors of evil, fear, legislation against certain activities and adoption of unfounded preventative measures. In 1977, when the media machine had engaged with HIV/AIDS, Susan Sontag, the famous American writer, film-maker and political activist, wrote

> ...illness is not a metaphor, and that the most truthful way of regarding illness—and the healthiest way of being ill—is one most purified of, most resistant to, metaphoric thinking.[40]

Reactions in the media

In the case of ME, the initial reaction in the 1990s has already been described – leading to stigmatisation from the outset and this has stuck. Until the scientific community and governments accept an irrefutable biomedical diagnosis, the false assumption that ME is somehow linked to lifestyle, dysfunctional personality or a psychological predisposition to this type of illness, will continue. The damage done by the initial media coverage, and to some extent by comments from the scientific community is enormous. The media look for the next big headline, they seek a reaction, and a new disease or virus which has unknown origin and impact, provides a great opportunity for speculation and sensationalism.

Those people who develop the disease or virus become the victims not only of the illness, but also of the media representation of their illness.

This can prejudice opinions of friends, family, the wider public, the medical profession, government departments and private companies who need to deal with employee sickness rights, sickness benefits and medical insurance claims. However, the media can also raise awareness and shock politicians into action.

Over the last five years, though, patients and advocates have had the playing field levelled to some extent due to the increased usage

---

[40] Sontag S. (1977) *Illness as Metaphor*. Toronto: McGraw-Hill Ryerson

and functionality of social media.

Not only is more information disseminated far quicker but the accessibility of the information, and debate and discussions around any subject, means that patients have become empowered and able to form powerful lobbying blocks which has been able to counter the false impression being presented by the media.

The Let's Do It For ME[41] campaign was formed by three severely affected patients who used social media to publicise new and exciting ways of supporting Invest in ME Research in raising awareness and funding for research. Despite being unable to leave their homes they organised a unique network of supporters who formed campaigns, entirely online, and helped the charity initiate a foundation research programme at UEA/IFR. Apart from mobilising patient power in this way, as never done before, the Let's Do It For ME team gave hope and empowerment to hundreds of participants and other patients around the world.

Once a story is able to gather momentum then it is possible for any issue to grab the headlines in a far more dynamic way, and more in-depth coverage can follow to raise awareness, correct misunderstandings and explain the illness in a vocabulary accessible to the general public.

Language is a very powerful tool. In her book 'Once upon a virus: AIDS legends and vernacular risk perception'[42], medical anthropologist Diane Goldstein (2004) describes how the AIDS virus became a construct of the language used to describe the virus:

> [...] story and science are interrelated, interactive, and ultimately constitute each other. This is not to say that T cells,

---

[41] Let's Do It For Me - www.ldifme.org
[42] Goldstein, D. (2004) Once upon a virus: AIDS legends and vernacular risk perception. Logan: Utah State University Press

test tubes, and retroviruses don't exist but, rather, that the natural world and the cultural world share the burden of creating disease realities [...] since tradition is dynamic, these expressive forms reflect the changes in beliefs and attitudes that come in response to new scientific developments, new understandings of transmission patterns, public health education programs, media coverage, current events, and so forth. The traditions, however, do not simply follow a specific trajectory chosen by public health or other officials but rather reflect the processing of a vast quantity of different and sometimes competing messages, all affecting disease understandings."

With HIV/AIDS the speculation about how, when and where the disease originated ran riot over a long period of time. Also, rumours of who was spreading the disease and modes of transition became subject to misleading and sometimes preposterous suggestions. Goldstein explains the history and dissemination of false information:

Early jokes focused on the gay population and the association of AIDS with drugs, eventually incorporating other notions of risk groups. These initial jokes focused on what came to be known as the 4 Hs: Homosexuals, Heroin users, Hemophiliacs, and Haitians. Like most health folklore, they assigned the disease to a group understood as distant from the teller [...] the jokes changed as public health and public education became more refined, evolving in response to emerging understandings of the disease.

Media headlines identified a virus for 'Yuppie Flu' and sowed the seeds of misunderstanding and prejudicial reactions to those presenting with the symptoms of what we now know to be ME. The 'legend' started; the virus was seen to be a result of a particular lifestyle that afflicted, in particular, a mixture of ambitious, over stimulated, burned out, upwardly mobile professionals. The reputation formed at the outset of the disease has never been shaken off despite research and government policies undermining this initial interpretation. This is how the power of the media can deliver what now seems to be a metaphorical curse on the public's understanding of the disease.

Anger, confusion and controversy

Of course the criticism of scientists involved in treatment trials for ME are not the only ones. The Autism-MMR (Measles, Mumps, Rubella) vaccine controversy has also engendered fierce criticism from parents who believe their autistic children were victims of a vaccine that has been universally promoted as safe by the medical establishment and research into possibly links has been criticized, undermined and dismissed, much to the anger of campaign groups who hoped to prove that the onset of autism is a directly linked to the vaccine. Viruses have been the subject of legend, controversy, suspicion and conspiracy theories since first widespread outbreaks, such as influenza, began. In the case of ME, patients have become angry and frustrated due to endless research into management regimes with no support being given to research that helps understand the basics of the disease. Patients want to know hard facts about their disease. However, we believe that the situation for ME is now at a turning point due to the involvement of leading scientists in biomedical research to find answers.

The collective understanding of disease

Other illnesses that have suffered misinterpretation and cruel mishandling by the media include anorexia nervosa and bulimia. Anorexia came suddenly into the public eye in 1982 when the famous American singer, Karen Carpenter, died of the condition at the age of 32 years. Her fame and physical decline made the headlines around the world and raised the profile of anorexia in medical and political spheres. Anorexia is now well supported by governments with publicly funded clinics all over the UK, free counseling and support services and awareness training for health practitioners on a scale never seen by ME. The reason is perhaps the death of a celebrity followed by the realization this condition can kill – one in five die from complications resulting from anorexia during their lifetime. However, there has been the same focus on the search for psychological factors in diagnosis influencing strongly any follow up treatment. New research is looking at serotonin levels before and after the onset of anorexia and it appears that abnormal levels precede the onset of the condition. This would overturn the belief that anorexia is a priori a psychological illness resulting from personal relationship dysfunction.

Understanding anorexia has not been helped by public figures such as Dame Joan Bakewell, writing in national newspapers about the reasons why anorexia affects some young people, particularly young girls. Her interview with The Sunday Times, 13 March 2016, reveals an embarrassing ignorance about the large amount of psychological and biological research into the causes of anorexia. "I am alarmed by anorexia among young people, which arises presumably because they are preoccupied with being beautiful and healthy and thin". This type of unsubstantiated statement undermines the intellectual superiority and expertise of scientists who do not share the same platform to speak to the nation. As with ME, unguarded and uninformed expressions of opinion by a public figure can result in harmful misunderstanding of and lasting stigma for those who suffer from the illness. They should leave such commentary to the experts.

In the case of the eating disorder bulimia, the illness made headlines in 1992 on the publication of the biography of Princess Diana written by Andrew Morton. He revealed that she had suffered from the disease through much of the 1980s. Diana admitted to the author that she had struggled with bulimia for many years and had received specialist treatment. Following her revelation many other people came forward to finally admit that they had an eating disorder and sought help. Scientists took up the lead and further research moved away from the psychological explanation towards a more complex biological cause, which in many cases is offset by psychological or emotional factors. The reaction of the public to the publicity and consequent discourse surrounding eating disorders was, and has remained, generally sympathetic.

When Princess Diana held the hand of a patient with AIDS it did much to eradicate the view that was prevalent at the time, i.e. the passage of the AIDS virus depended on body contact. It is much more difficult to get celebrities with ME speaking up in the media in contrast to the many patients' stories of which we have included some examples in this book. Again, when a massive campaign on AIDS was launched by the Thatcher government in the UK there were serious political debates in the Cabinet about the extent to which the public posters should show the earthquake nature of the potential tragedies of getting AIDS. At the same time there were heated debates about associating such publicity with the sexual mores of the times. Effects on young people were to be ignored lest it encouraged certain practices.

This collective understanding of a disease can create a whole new set of relationships in families, friendship groups, communities, workplace and in society generally. Some of these relationships may be positive and supportive whilst others prove to be negative and those who are afflicted by the disease may suffer rejection, be forgotten, ignored or in the worst of cases, ridiculed. Alliances are formed with those professionals who take on the issues surrounding the disease in different spheres – political, medical, scientific fields and as carers, or in financial and legal roles. The disease generates a whole new set of collaborations between those who have a disease and those who find themselves involved at some level. The many ME support groups and charities have become a vehicle for involving different actors and giving a platform for the patients to express their own opinions, hopes, feelings and frustrations.

Culture and disease

Anthropologists sometimes refer to culture-bound syndromes where physical symptoms are bound up with psychological disorders. However, some anthropologists, such as Anthony Wallace[43], have challenged this view and see the disease commencing with a physical disorder due to environment or metabolic deficiencies that develop neurological and psychological symptoms. The concept of 'somatisation', where a psychological disorder or stress is expressed through physical symptoms, still holds fast in the minds of many medical practitioners, leading to false diagnosis and treatment. Only a deeper understanding of the physiology of the symptoms of ME will move people away from the prevalence of psychological explanations. The best research combines biochemical factors with social and environmental factors. "Without neuroendocrinological data, anthropologists are unable to study the biochemical pathways that may lead to mental illness, addiction and culture-bound syndromes"[44] which equally

---

[43] Wallace, Anthony (1972) Mental Illness, Biology and Culture in *Psychological Anthropology* pp362-402.
[44] McElroy, A. and Townsend, P. (2009) *Medical Anthropology in Ecological Perspective*. Colorado: Westview Press.

applies to ME.

There are many different voices that frame and inform public opinion in relation to ME. There are the voices of scientists agreeing and disagreeing, politicians urging or dismissing pleas from victims and carers to act, the voices of bureaucracies talking of rules, rights, requirements, assessments and diagnoses. Then there are the voices of the victims themselves, their friends and relatives. These are the voices that are seldom heard outside the support groups. Their language is about abandonment, wasted lives, loss, being forgotten and misunderstood. It is a language of desperation in many cases and expressed through websites, blogs, YouTube, emails and online forums. Just do an internet search on ME (or ME/CFS, or CFS, or CFS/ME) and page after page appears from those suffering from ME where they share stories and experiences, give advice and warnings.

When those afflicted by ME talk to medical practitioners, employers, insurance companies, social security assessors, the language they use to describe their symptoms is crucial to the diagnosis and interpretation of their illness. They have no official representation in the medical hierarchy of government and few politicians take up their cause and elevate it to the public platform. The names of celebrities who suffer from ME do not make news in the same way that those with AIDS, drug, alcohol or painkiller addictions do. The list of those who have had HIV/AIDS or life threatening addictions is long and well known – Boy George, Paula Yates, Michael Jackson, Keith Moon, Freddie Mercury, Dean Martin – to name just a few.

So are there no celebrities with ME?

There are, but news of their illness has not been well publicized. Celebrities who are known or rumoured to have/have had ME include Publicist and writer Howard Bloom, Stevie Nicks of the band Fleetwood Mac, film directors Blake Edwards and David Puttnam, actor Michael Crawford, yachtswoman Clare Francis and also, famously, the singer Cher. In 1992, Cher took some time off from her career. She was reported as saying that she caught a virus, the Epstein Barr virus, which later turned out to be ME, and "Boy, it was devastating for me...I wasn't able to work for almost three years".

Yet these celebrity cases did not result in the political attention and action one would have expected. The term 'the forgotten ones' rings true for those with ME. Due to the influence of the biopsychosocial model and those who promote it there continues to be the misunderstanding and misinterpretation of ME at all levels of society that is still going on despite official confirmation by government bodies worldwide that the condition is neurological not psychological? This question undermines the whole issue. As recently as 2015, the IOM (Institute of Medicine) in the USA has announced that

> myalgic encephalomyelitis (ME) and chronic fatigue syndrome (CFS) are serious, debilitating conditions that affect millions of people in the United States and around the world [...] it is a medical - not a psychiatric or psychological – illness [...] without a known cause or effective treatment which can cause significant impairment and disability" rendering 25% of patients homebound or bedridden.

They also declare that "the term chronic fatigue syndrome can result in trivialization and stigmatization" of this "complex, multisystem, and often devastating disorder.[45]

---

[45] Committee on the Diagnostic Criteria for Myalgic Encephalomyelitis/Chronic Fatigue Syndrome, Board on the Health of

And yet many doctors remain ignorant of the disease and its classification since 1969 by the World Health Organization as a neurological disease. Having consulted recent graduates of medicine it seems they have received little or no education about ME apart from rudimentary diagnostic criteria (see Chapter 2).

Is this a blatant case of politicians and health care providers and educators uniting against the reality of a widespread and devastating disease? As with most contested areas of health, the financial implication of supporting, researching and compensating those afflicted is the most likely explanation for relegating the disease to the realms of a psychological disorder which can be fixed by self-help exercise regimes and a bit of counseling. Indeed, this is the same tragic conclusion reached by George Faulkner in his 2016 report for the Centre for Welfare Reform entitled 'In the Expectation of Recovery':

Dubious claims of biopsychosocial expertise have been used to serve the interests of influential institutions and individuals in government, medical research and the insurance industry, where concerns about money and reputation will inevitably compete with concerns about public health and patients' rights.[46]

Economic recession in the West has meant that government spending on biomedical research has increasingly been forced to compete with other areas of the economy. The emergence of new infectious diseases – Ebola, SARS, Zika - demanded urgent research funding. It is partly for this reason that ME has not received the attention and investment in research needed to make real progress. Instead patchwork solutions and temporary fixes have been offered, but these are not serious interventions to target the disease and prevent further cases developing.

Select Populations, Institute of Medicine (2015) *Beyond Myalgic Encephalomyelitis* (Washington DC): National Academies Press (US).
[46] www.centreforwelfarereform.org

In the next chapter we shall look at research under way today and what hope there is for the future.

Lost Voices from a Hidden Illness

There are so many tragic stories about ME. The book Lost Voices from a Hidden Illness[47] describes the experiences of 32 very different people who have ME and the effect it has had on their lives, family and friends. It was commissioned as a project to collect these individual stories by the charity Invest in ME Research (IiMER). The charity listed its objective as "making a change in how ME is perceived and treated in the media, by health departments and by healthcare professionals. We aim to do this by identifying the three key areas to concentrate our efforts on - funding for biomedical research, education and lobbying. Invest in ME Research aims to collaborate and coordinate events and activities in these areas in order to provide the focus and funding to allow biomedical research to be carried out."[48]

I met recently with Richard and Pia Simpson who are a driving force behind IiMER. Their own story is one of ongoing struggle. Richard and Pia continue to support their two daughters who both developed ME from their early teenage years. They fight to get recognition of the disease from the medical establishment, to challenge existing ineffective treatments and find alternative biomedical treatments, play a vital role in sourcing research funding and keeping ME on the political agenda. I leave you with the words of Richard Simpson in Lost Voices as he describes the impact of ME on his family as he and his wife Pia fight to find a cure for their daughters from the illness with no quick fix, largely

---

[47] Boulton, N. (ed.) (2010) *Lost Voices from a Hidden Illness.* Wild Conversations Press
[48] www.investinme.org (accessed 25.5.2016)

ignored and widely misunderstood.

> We were ill-prepared for this illness. Ill-prepared to discover how little help there was to treat it or cope with it, let alone cure it, and how the basic infrastructure of society fails the citizens they are meant to support. Ill-prepared for the isolation that would pervade our daughters' lives. (p59)

> Everything is reduced – we adapt and learn to cope and reduce our expectations – of friends, of family, of healthcare services, of politicians, of this society. ME rules our lives……. We see what could be done to provide a cure for this illness if the will and the morality were applied to treating ME. (p60)

After the IIMEC11 conference in London in 2016, one comment showed how inclusive the occasion was for the views of charities, carers and counselors alike. Referring to Ian Gibson's chairmanship of the conference the attendee wrote:

> *It was your manner and your words which ensured that folk like me (in 67 years, that was my first experience of a science-connected event) could feel included; to ensure that we all felt we had permission to ask questions, to talk to the speakers at the intervals; and perhaps most important of all, that we left the hall at the end of that long day with hope…*

The strength of our campaign ultimately depends on the various factions working together and not against each other.

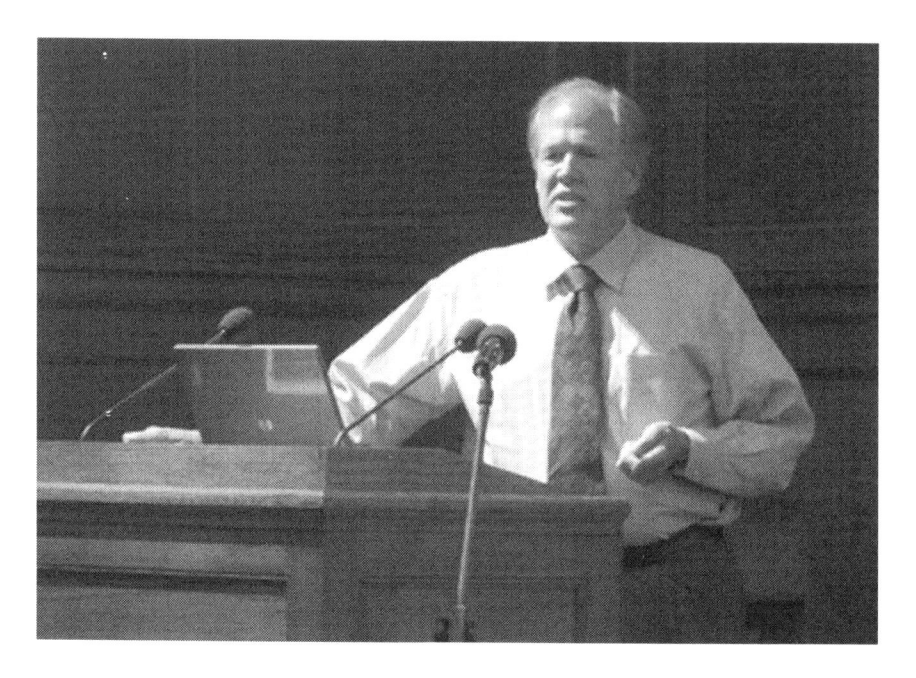

Dr Dan Peterson (above) and Professor Malcolm Hooper (below) at an Invest in ME Research International ME Conference

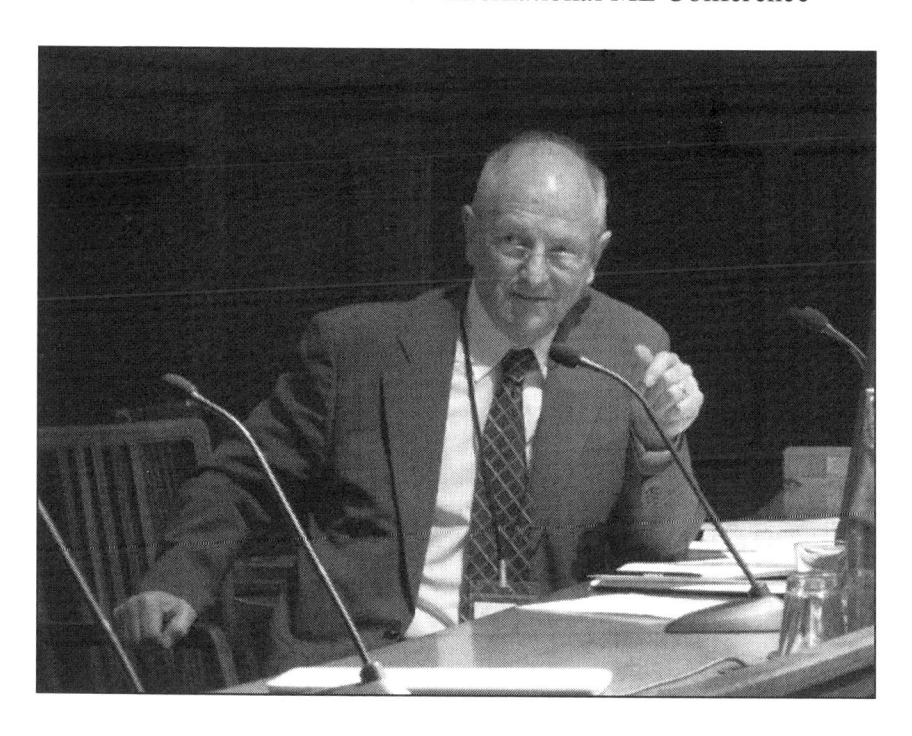

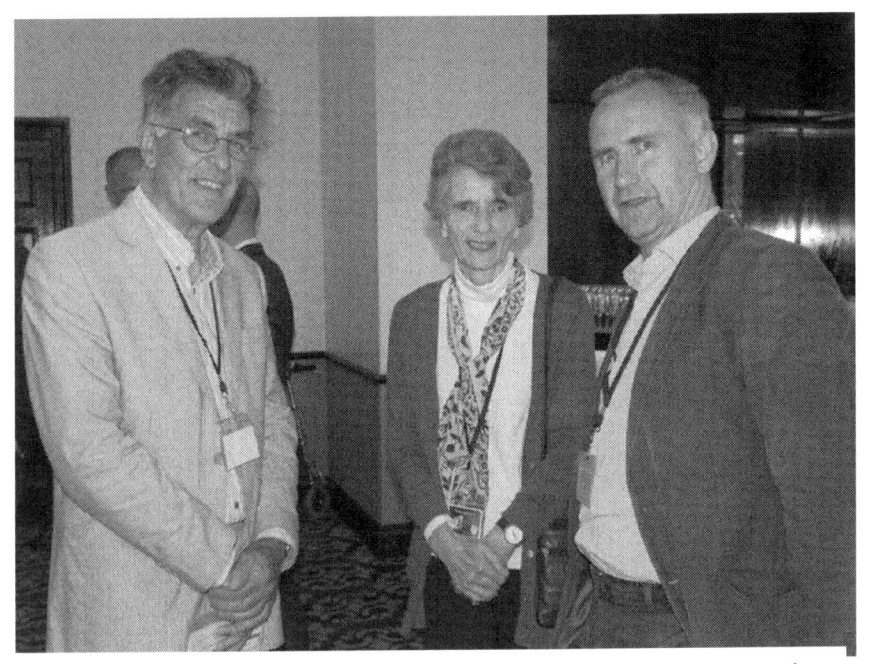

Above: Professor Jonathan Edwards (UCL), Professor Angela Vincent (Oxford University) and Dr Neil Harrison (Sussex University) at an Invest in ME Research International Colloquium.
Below: Countess of Mar and Dr Nigel Speight at an Invest in ME Research pre-conference dinner

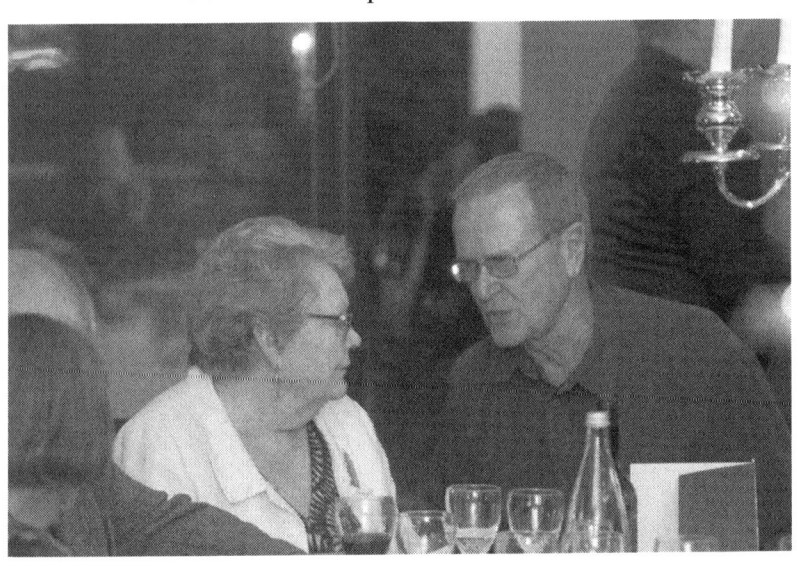

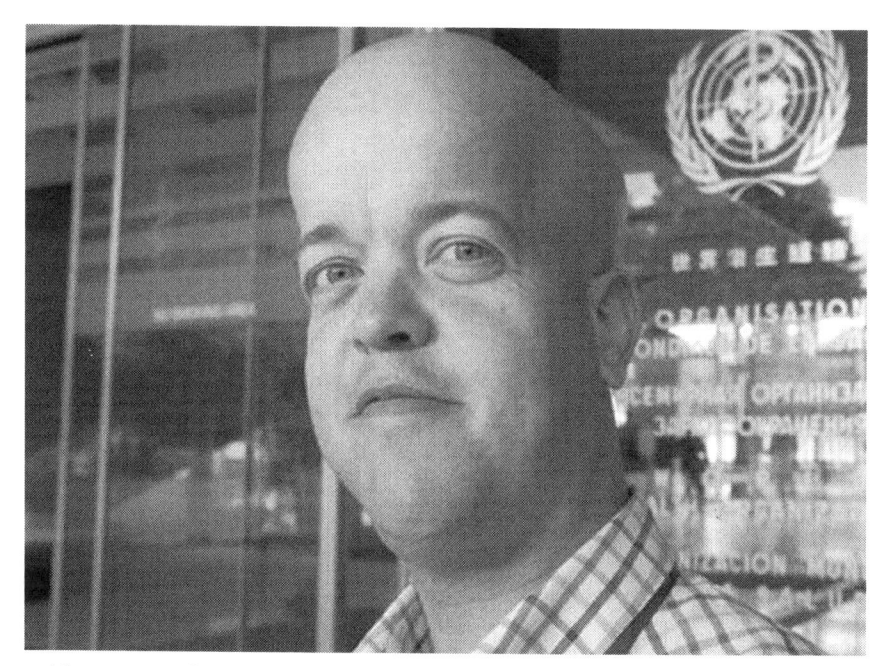

Above: Professor Tom Shakespeare (University of East Anglia).
Below: Fane Mensah and Dr Geraldine Cambridge (UCL, UK)

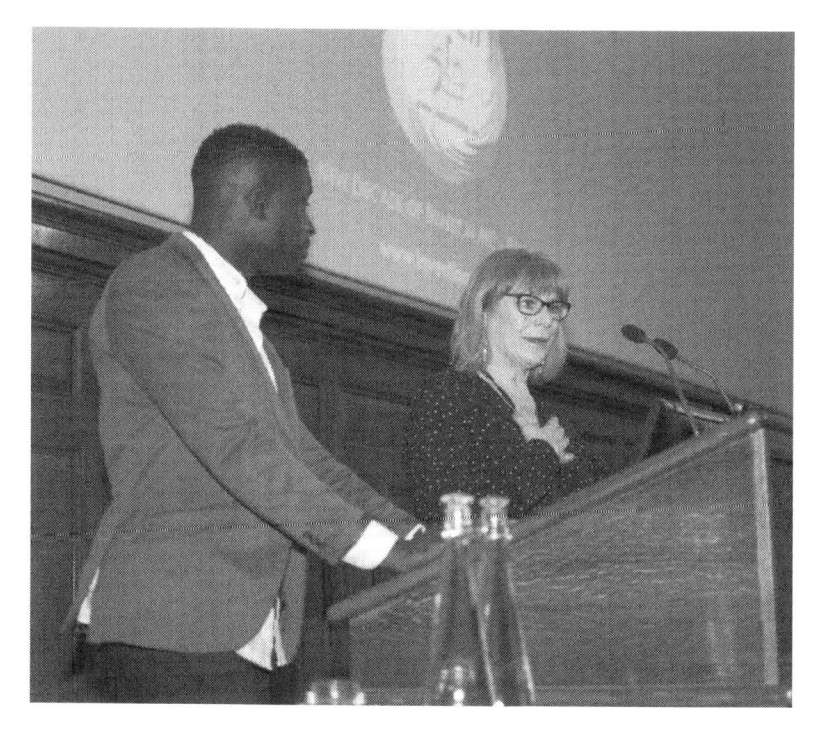

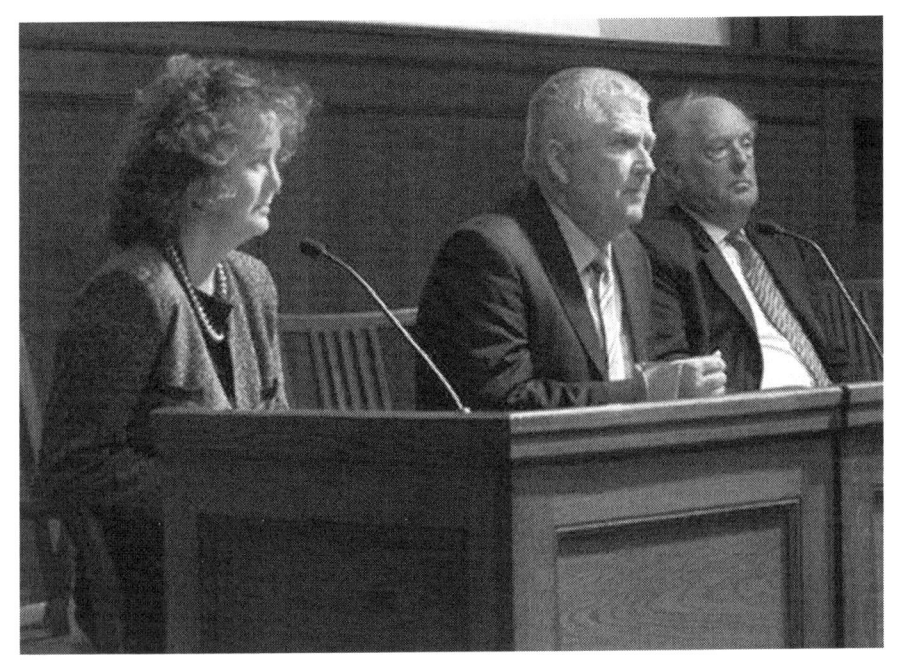

Above: Professor Sonya Marshall-Gradisnik and Professor Don Staines (NCNED, Griffiths University, Australia)

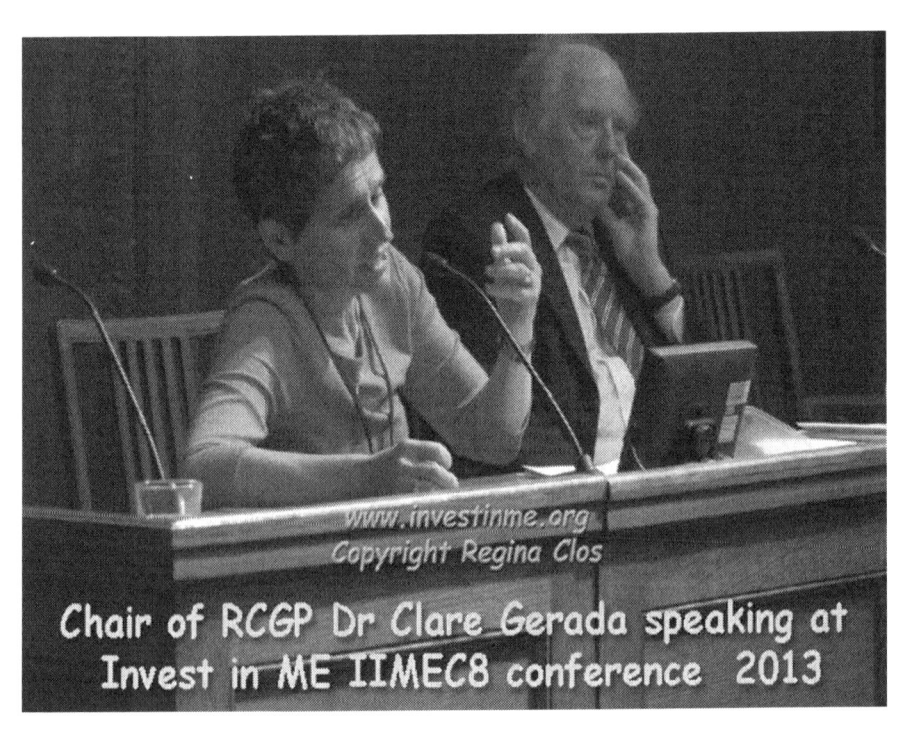

Chair of RCGP Dr Clare Gerada speaking at Invest in ME IIMEC8 conference 2013

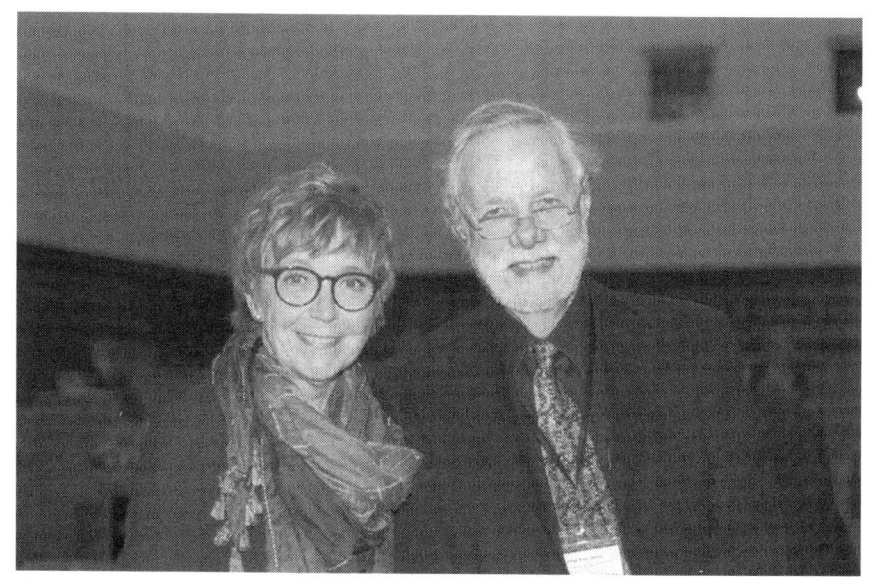

Above: Kjersti Krisner from Norway and Professor Ron Davis (Stanford Genome Technology Center, USA)
Below: Associate Professor Mady Hornig (Columbia University, USA) and Dr Vicky Whittemore (National Institutes of Health, USA)

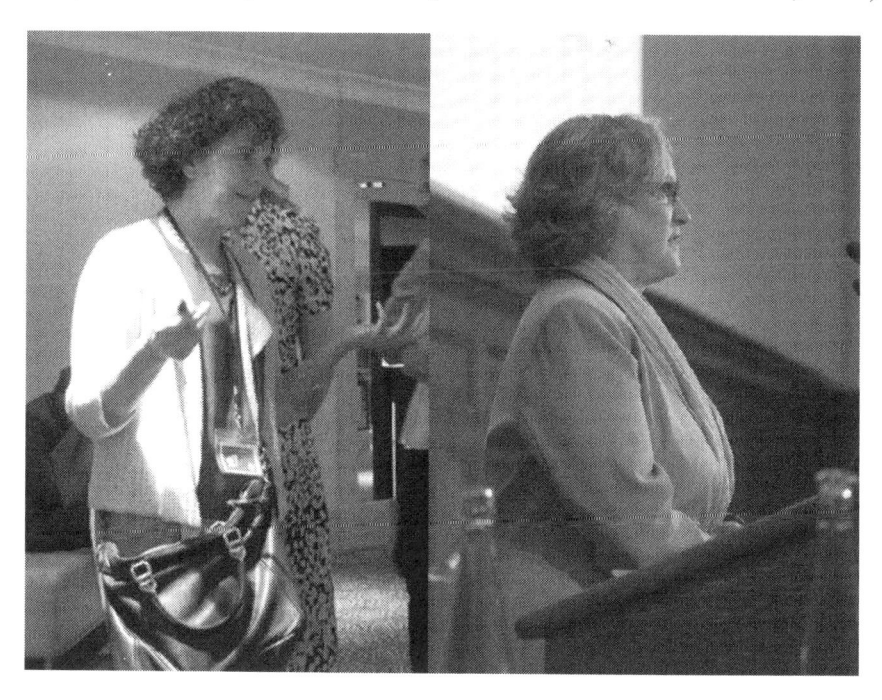

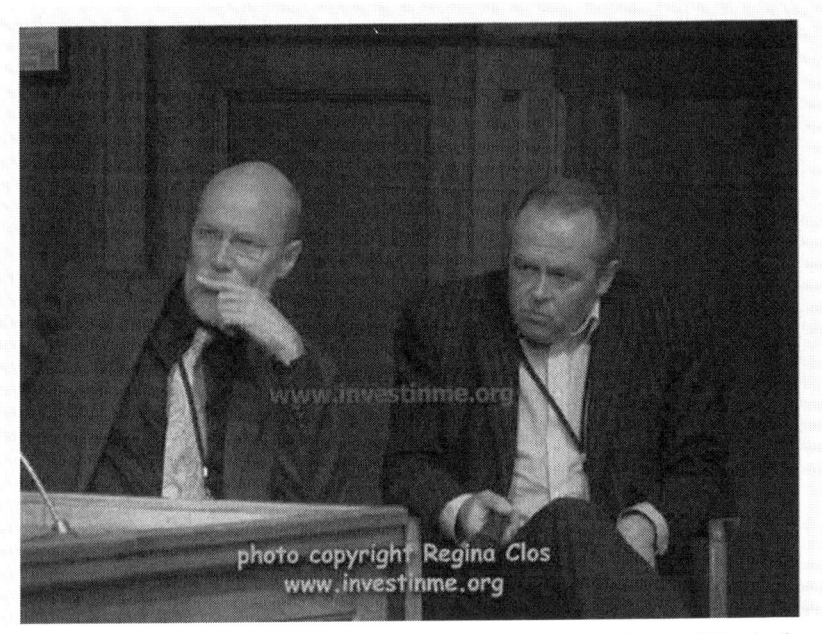

Above: Professor Olav Mella and Dr Øystein Fluge (Haukeland University Hospital, Bergen. Below: The UEA/IFR group – Professor Simon Carding, Professor Tom Wileman and author Dr Ian Gibson

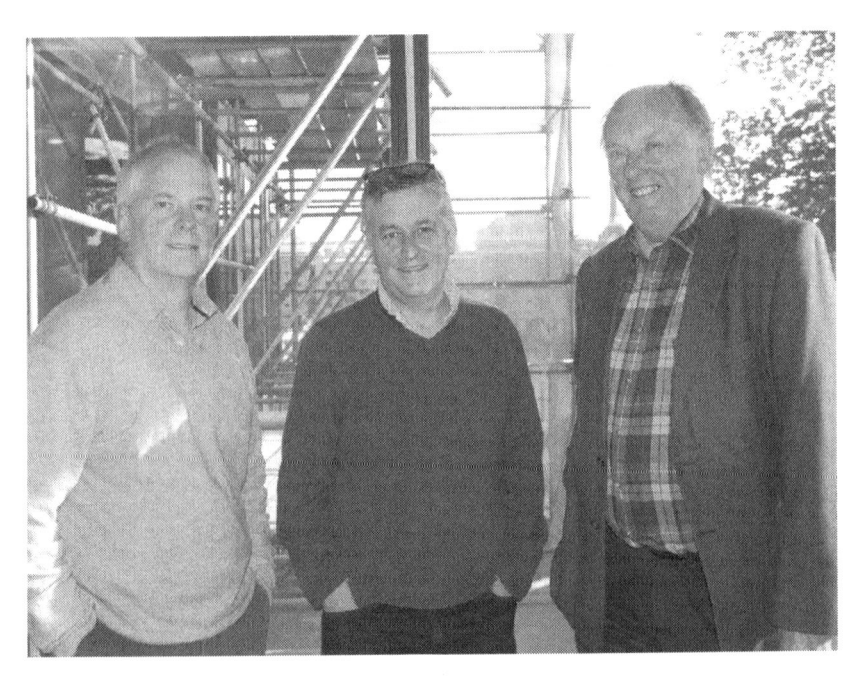

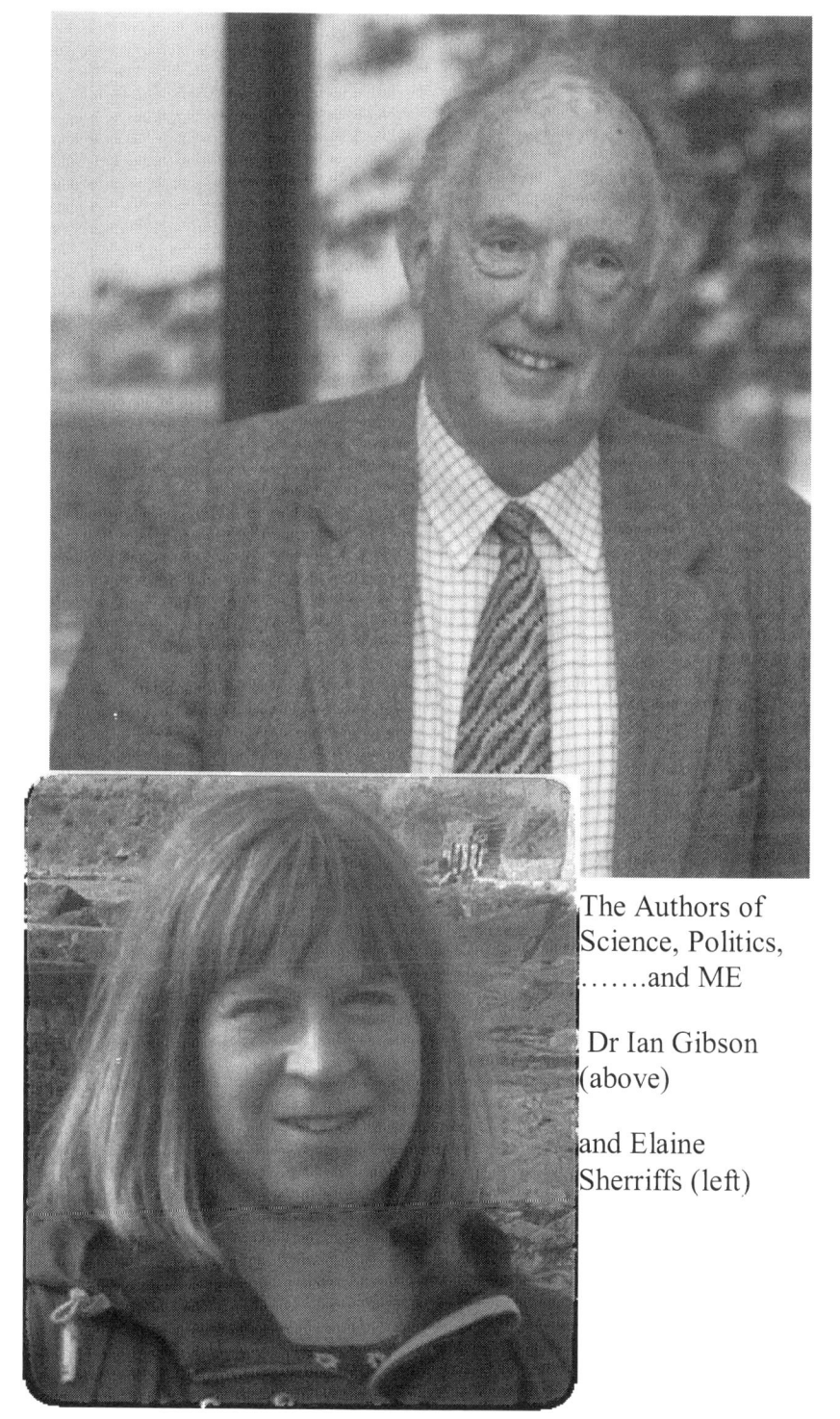

The Authors of Science, Politics, …….and ME

Dr Ian Gibson (above)

and Elaine Sherriffs (left)

Chapter 4 - The Politics of it All

Introduction

Much of what has been written about ME and the research into its causes ignores the broader discussion of the National Health Service in the UK. Currently there is a debate on how much its aim of providing a free service at the point of need is being eroded by privatisation of various services within a health provision for all of the people. It is an imperative that we consider the trends in the health spending on research, care and treatment if we are to realistically address the funding for ME. Will there ever be enough finance provided to tackle such an illness? Indeed, the availability of monies for the illnesses associated with viruses in Africa e.g. Ebola, and the Zika virus has depended on an international programme involving contributions from many countries including the United Nations. The criteria often used in the debates around the programmes were that the illness must at least be an international health crisis. Officials jump into action if it threatens the spread across national borders. Epidemics and their spread across the globe are unpredictable.

Some readers will see that ME also fulfils certain uncertainties but there is no evidence, it is said, that it kills numbers of people to the same extent as viruses like Ebola – 11,000 in a short period of time – or is associated with the development of microcephaly in children. Clearly there will always be reasons to put the problem of ME in a lower league if you only use certain criteria. The question arises, however, when to elevate the illness to the higher league and take steps to address a cure or at least slow down the advance of the illness in the individual and the population. Many are convinced that the time has come to recognise the seriousness of the condition and that many of the arguments about defining the illness or its causes pales in the need for recognition of the patients and carers who see for themselves the effects on individuals. In fact, like cancer, everybody seems to know someone with ME. Even in the cancer field certain cancers receive priority attention and we have even seen the evolution of the term 'rare cancers' that justifies a lower priority in terms of medical initiatives.

It is then argued that as medical technology and treatments move on that political priorities change. Whilst this is clearly true as new drugs and new surgical methods are developed there remains the burning question of who decides on the priorities and indeed should there be any. New illnesses arrive on the world scene or locally for many reasons to do with new environments, new foods, changes in climate, new biological entities or whatever and we really should be ready and able to react to these. These events may arrive in a short period of time or over longer periods. The movement of insects carrying deadly viruses or the advent of biological weapons should be taken seriously and a rapid response unit be made ready. If, however, you deny there is an illness, as with ME, then nothing will be done. The history of ME tells us that it was never taken seriously as an illness with a biological basis and that it was alleged to be a psychiatric illness.

The cry of more money for the Health Service is reverberating around our islands in 2016. Money without proper direction and serious management which uses or seeks to make decisions based on clinical or scientific evidence can lead to failures in diagnosis, treatments and care programmes. Campaigns calling today for more money are challenged to identify priorities which they often seem unwilling to do and particularly in issues around mental health and dementia, autism, ME, multiple sclerosis, diabetes etc. etc. As Aneurin Bevin pointed out in the early 20th Century, it is often associated with the argument that the NHS is a bottomless pit. The argument then proceeds to paying for your health care from cradle to grave. The alternative view is to recognise that all illnesses deserve proper funding from the Exchequer and to encourage proper and careful use of these funds. A current piece of research shows one way forward for the argument of increasing health service funding in relation to the growth of countries in Europe.

Many voices have been raised over the years about Gross Domestic Product (GDP) being used as an economic indicator. They include many eminent economists like Joseph Stiglitz, politicians like Robert Kennedy, Jose Barroso and David Cameron who all call for 'moving beyond the gross domestic product as our main measure of progress' and call on us to fashion a 'sustainable development index that puts people first.' (UN General Bank: Moon, 2012).

Despite all the honeyed words, and it is hard to find a politician who has not said something about GDP, and for all the talk of environmental challenges, quality of life and distributional aspects of income, nothing is given to ME patients. The world does not move on in the face of powerful voices advocating the use of GDP measures e.g. Paul Samuelson, Robert McNamara who agree how this measurement has 'contributed significantly to exacerbate the inequalities of income distribution'.

I was once told by an eminent member of the Clinical Commissioning Group in Norwich that I could 'sing for it' (the money) if I was asking for financial support to take care of ME patients and to provide a local consultant who prioritised the condition in some of the clinics.

The current demands for more money into the UK National Health Service for better care and research at presentation of illness, have not been addressed by our current government. The UK is spending less in comparison with other countries in Europe. By 2020 £43 billion would need to be injected into the budget if we are to equalise the proportion of the Gross Domestic Product with 12 other European countries.

A letter to The Guardian newspaper on 2 February 2016 from Professor Colin Pritchard (School of Health & Social Care, Bournemouth University and Visiting Professor, Department of Psychiatry, University of Southampton)[49] points out that according the World Bank (2013) the UK spends only 9.1% of GDP on health, compared to the European average of 10.3%. Indeed, our EU partners spend 11.6% (France) and 11.3% (Germany) whilst the USA spends 17.1%.

Amongst Western nations the UK comes 18th out of 21 countries for the percentage of GDP spent on health services. John Appleby, Chief Economist of The King's Fund, an independent charity working to improve health and care in England, is quoted in the same paper warning that Britain's continued low spending on health care will mean that any improvements planned in the quality of care and outcomes from treatment will not be delivered. This failure to keep pace with the amount other nations spends on healthcare means the UK will slide even further down the international league tables.

Norman Lamb, MP for North Norfolk and health minister in the Conservative-Liberal Democrat coalition government, advises us "The NHS and care systems will crash if we carry on as we are because the amount [going into the NHS] is not enough and everyone in the NHS knows it". [50]

However, we measure the input required for the NHS, Appleby and his team agree that we need to compare with the best in

---

[49] The Guardian. Letters. Tuesday 2 February 2016.
[50] The Guardian. *'UK is falling behind on NHS funding'*. Page 2, 20 January 2016.

Europe, i.e. France and Germany. The current Conservative government congratulates itself on ring fencing the NHS budget, increasing its share of government spending and financial annual boosts to £8.4 billion by 2020-21. Figures are tossed around by politicians but there is no denying that £43 billion is necessary to match other European standards. As UK GDP is forecast to grow by 15.2% from 2014-2021, NHS spending will fail to reflect this increase.

As pointed out by Turner and Gibson[51], in 2000 Labour's then Prime Minister, Tony Blair, promised to increase spending in the NHS to the European average of 8.5% of GDP, which Gordon Brown eventually agreed to and delivered in 2009. It was drawn out from him by the astute questioning of one David Frost on a Sunday morning political programme. Labour was committed to meet the EU average of the proportionate share of rising GDP. However, neither the Labour party nor the Tory party are willing to commit in 2016 to increasing health care costs to meet the current European average of 10.1%. Thus the gap between Britain and its European counterparts continues to widen as the country fails to keep pace with international spending. The effects of the BREXIT decision on research and, eventually, healthcare are also unknowns at this time.

Given this lack of commitment and political will, in the absence of a public revolt or by adopting new financial methodologies of funding the NHS it does not augur well for a commitment to tackling research into ME, particularly biomedical. In the face of a fascination with psychiatric research and a belief that this is where the treatments will emerge, it looks even more remote a possibility. The PACE Trial investigation, where £5 million was given for its operation, has made many people suspicious that a full research

---

[51] Turner, D. and Gibson I. (2013) 'Best When We Are Labour?' Brighton: Pen Press Publications.

programme will never occur, given the research climate. It is necessary to recognise that excellent research is being undertaken in well-equipped laboratories by well-trained scientists and medical personnel, usually supported by private money. It is time for the state funding bodies to realise that no longer can they argue that there are no good projects on the research agenda. Some of these use molecular techniques and approaches that are beginning to produce interesting results. The time is ripe for new attitudes to funding and support for new ideas and hypotheses. The current research programmes are outlined in Chapter 2, but the necessary funding is short of what is needed for an adequate research programme. Sometimes, too, serendipitous, unrelated research turns out to be relevant for some other illness other than the one which is favoured for support.

How Things Started - the Kevin Short Connection

But before entering these areas of current interest let us point out how one of the authors (Ian Gibson) became involved in this field of endeavour. Ian was introduced to ME through an individual in Norwich, Kevin Short, who asked Ian to visit him and talk over his problems.

Kevin Short lived in Norwich in 2005. He phoned to ask if Ian would come and visit him to talk about his illness. Ian was hooked. The challenge of taking up such an issue was too much. Over a time in Parliament since 1997 he had learned how certain illnesses were popular with governments and the Department of Health. Ian had led a campaign on improving cancer services and was now taking up mental health issues given the huge challenges. As a Health Charity Champion in the House of Commons for 3 years in a row Ian felt confident in taking up a health issue in London. There had been a debate on ME in the 1st Parliament since the election of a Labour Government in 1997. Tony Wright, the MP for Great Yarmouth, had set up an active All Party Group on ME. Norfolk connections with a local charity had drawn Ian into the group that he eventually chaired.

The Gibson Inquiry

At the time that Ian met Kevin Short (who had formed a group called Anglia ME Action), he was a Member of Parliament for Norwich North. About the same time Ian visited 3 constituents, all with ME, who found it difficult to 'get up' and had weak muscles, fatigue and several other problems. They recounted the difficulty of convincing their General Practitioners that they were ill. Ian met patients in his constituency office who were knowledgeable of their illness but hugely disappointed by the poor treatment centres in Norfolk. He promised to set up an inquiry in Parliament using his experience as former Chair of the House of Commons Select Committee on Science and Technology. Ian was also a 'Champion for Health', Backbencher of the Year and very active in many health problems. This had taken him into national and international policy making as well as scientific meetings.

Having met all the charities in the UK, and Invest in ME Research that included people in Norwich, Richard and Pia Simpson, the latter asked Ian to speak at their international conference in London. Since that time Ian has missed only 1 or 2 in the past 11 years. Following the inquiry report the charity asked Ian to chair their international meeting and since then he has, through attending it, met charities, scientists, politicians in other countries and reporters who expressed interest in tackling the cruel symptoms of this condition.

An inquiry was unlike a Select Committee study but there were similarities. A group was set up (see below) with the help of Tony

Wright's employee who offered to take the minutes and bring witnesses. The minutes can be viewed online, as can much of what witnesses said. The report came out in November 2006.[52] Major events inducing Ian to set it up were further visits to some of his constituents who were bed-bound and visits from Professor Malcolm Hooper and a GP, Terry Mitchell, who ran an ME clinic in Great Yarmouth.

The Gibson Inquiry, whilst it drew criticism from some regarding its significance, its availability, its administrative failure to make research and treatment monies to be widely available etc., was still considered a success in many people's eyes. It was a take-off point in the approach of many for ME and attracted favourable comment. Support was drawn from the elected and non-elected Houses and were friends of Ian's who were bright, interested and who contributed time for free. There were no payments to any of those involved as it was done alongside the many other activities of parliamentarians. Thanks must go to Richard Taylor MP, Ann Cryer MP, Michael Meacher MP, Des Turner MP, David Taylor MP and Lord Turnberg, the Countess of Mar and Baroness Cumberlege. They were superb and their support and any political differences were evidently irrelevant. Sadly, we have recently lost both Michael Meacher and David Taylor.

Shrill responses came from a few individuals who said the minutes were sparse; the secretary left Parliament half way through the proceedings, that the inquiry had no parliamentary status and the Chair was in the pocket of the pharmaceutical industry. This was the best of the criticism. The inquiry did have an effect on the Invest in ME Research charity, which picked up the cudgels particularly where it said that equal support, financial or other, should go to those who believed in a biomedical explanation.

---

[52] http://www.erythos.com/gibsonenquiry/Report.html

Since then the battle has continued on the basis of forgetting the few critics and developing a research programme. The Norwich team met regularly to advance this aim. The report attracted the interest of the Minister of Health, Andy Burnham and many major players to tackle the problem. This seems a long time ago at this moment. There was a press conference given where spokespeople representing other charities and even the government sought to discredit the report. There were some sparse positive statements in the inquiry. Margaret Williams, a formidable ME activist, said:

> Whilst there will be some people who may be disappointed that more weight was not given to the wealth of existing biomedical evidence, the UK ME/CFS community owes a debt of gratitude to Dr Ian Gibson MP and to most of his committee members for agreeing to tackle such an immensely complicated issue. It is a remarkable achievement that, considering the difficulties under which they laboured (especially the total lack of funding) and the opposition that they faced, they have produced such a valuable Report that must surely help to move matters forwards in the direction that will best support and help – and not damage – patients who have been so abused for so long.

Professor Hooper concluded:

> Dr Gibson and his Inquiry team are to be congratulated on their report and the splendid work of his voluntary Parliamentary research staff deserves a warm vote of thanks for their efforts that brought this demanding Inquiry to such a satisfactory conclusion. Well done everyone [.....] Only a full Government Inquiry can address all these issues satisfactorily and this must be established as advocated by the Gibson Inquiry.

The period following the Gibson Inquiry

The report was published in 2006 by members of both Houses of the UK Parliament. The minister at the time dodged the major thrust of the discussions by merely saying that no good applications had been received for biomedical research grants by the Medical Research Council (MRC). This helped justify the grants that were given by the MRC which were criticised as mainly responding to the psychiatric lobby which centered around certain universities – King's College London, Bristol and QMUL, for example. There was deep bitterness within large sectors of the ME interest groups and some of this spilled over into a criticism of the Inquiry despite the concentration in its conclusions on the need for biomedical research alongside the psychiatric approaches. This was of course understandable when one group was seen to be dominating research funding pathways and also media campaigns.

As an example we can look at an article penned by The Guardian journalist writing as a freelance in the Lancet, 2011. The article by Nigel Hawkes was entitled 'Dangers of research into chronic fatigue syndrome'[53], tackled claims of aggressive attacks on doctors and academics, in particular Sir Simon Wessely of Kings College School of Medicine. The people were described by Professor Wessely as 'sulphurous, vicious, horrible' (2011:p1). They attacked the PACE Trial and its results and whilst one or two individuals may have overstepped the mark this was drowned out by serious complaints and criticisms by other scientists and medical personnel who knew what they were talking about. Many journalists did not enter the debate due to the atmosphere and some raised the complaint that research was being hindered whatever the approach – psychiatric or biomedical – by this situation.
Following the NICE report on potential treatments for ME, High

---

[53] Hawkes, Nigel (2011). 'Dangers of research into chronic fatigue syndrome'. BMJ 2011;342:d3780

Court action ensued and reputations were maligned it was claimed. Academics and scientists retreated from the fray.

There was a similar reaction to some MPs after the 2006 Gibson Inquiry. Individuals who supported the conclusions were pilloried in their MP's surgeries. In fact, a very senior member of the Inquiry wished to withdraw his name over the report since it-might affect his relationship with other members of the Royal College of Physicians and no doubt his personal friendships. He was persuaded not to and he did eventually progress to becoming a government minister.

There was, however, movement behind the scenes by the MRC and the Department of Health no doubt with the knowledge of government ministers since new studies were set up with the MRC and money offered on the basis of 'good research' and the incorporation of a scientist on the team who had not directly been involved in ME research before. This was, of course, meant to take care of the bias seen by the patient group in the selection of funding committee members. One very positive response to the Inquiry was from UK charity Invest in ME Research who found it to be of value in nurturing research locally in Norwich at a local research institute.

Suffice it to say there was no open response from the government and civil servants to the Gibson Inquiry but it was not surprising since even Select Committee reports get little or no response from an official committee in terms of actions and acknowledgement for being a good policy initiative.

What members of the committee went through was similar to the attitude of the medical establishment in the USA to the events and 'epidemic' at Incline Village and their reaction to the two doctors who identified the problem of ME and were pilloried for it locally and nationally by politicians and the medical establishment. I have no doubt the Department of Health in the UK were acting and attacking the committee as well confirming the irrelevance of ME. The Committee persisted despite administrative problems with the production of minutes as the administrator moved on to more lucrative work with a political ally and there was little encouragement from officials, politicians or even patient groups. The isolation of the Committee of Inquiry as an 'unofficial' group is a political tactic which the members of the Inquiry group were aware of.

The Gibson Inquiry report was sent to all MPs in the House of Commons, relevant Ministers and Senior Medical and other scientific figures for review. In early December the report had been sent to Andy Burnham, the then Minister for Health in the Labour Government, for review.

On 21 December 2006 a covering letter was sent with the report by the author, Dr Ian Gibson as Chair of the Group on Scientific Research into Chronic Fatigue Syndrome/Myalgic Encephalomyelitis, to government ministers. Excerpts from the letter are below:

Over the past year this group has conducted an Inquiry into the issues surrounding CFS/ME. I attach a copy of the Inquiry's Report for you to review.

There are some 250,000 people suffering from CFS/ME in the UK, yet we have fallen behind the rest of the world when it comes to researching and recognising a biomedical model of the illness. The only treatments available to patients are symptomatic and there has been no major scientific research into its causes on a national level. This is despite the fact that CFS/ME is now five times more prevalent in the UK than AIDS and can be just as debilitating. The Group feels that this issue must be addressed.

The Report calls for massive investment into and commissioning of biomedical research projects. The Group found that in the UK there has been a historical bias towards funding research into the psychosocial model of the illness. This model is contradicted by work in Canada, the US and Australia. The Group is concerned for patients who at present are only offered symptomatic treatments and can find it extremely difficult to get the recognition or benefits they need from government. We are concerned that the UK appears to be falling behind the rest of the world when it comes to research and innovation in this area.

In addition, more radically, the letter urges future research to exclude the psychological approach. The Report also calls for an independent panel made up of virologists, immunologists, biochemists, endocrinologists, geneticists to review the international and UK biomedical evidence to identify areas for future research. This panel should exclude psychiatrists and psychologists and be independent of the existing CFS/ME debate.

The main thrust of the letter was to initiate funding based on the conclusions of the report:

The Group urges you to read our report and look into establishing proper funding for research in this area. We have an unprecedented opportunity to make a real difference to patients' lives and to give the illness the recognition it deserves.

After publication of the report and a press conference it is true to say that only the Mail on Sunday took it up and published a serious critique in its Journal after an interview with the Chairman. Other newspapers and journals ran for cover and felt it was all too hot to handle. One or two Department of Health officials privately told Ian it was a no-go area of research and to be careful of saying too much.

Around this time Ian had been invited to discussions on the setting up of a Science Media Centre from meetings with Baroness Greenfield at the Royal Institution. This was in the aftermath of the genetically modified crop issue in 1998 where scientists were very poor or worse at convincing the public. So a structure was set up to give 'establishment' scientists and institutions or departments a voice and access to the media. In the field of ME this has mainly been used to give the psychiatric lobby on ME an introduction to mass communication following conferences. Interestingly, Professor Simon Wessely is a trustee of the organisation. Much has been written about the organisation's funding. At about the same time a group 'Sense about Science' was set up by Lord Taverne, a Liberal Democrat peer to ensure that evidence based science help sway in policy making. This, of course, makes the right noises but in the experience of the authors fails to understand how science is practised and how today's hypothesis becomes true or is replaced following further investigations.

Their talks are punctuated by the belief that there is one truth and it is irreplaceable. This is obviously true at any one moment until the next programme of research. The scientific 'mind' keeps its options open. Scientists who also think about the political implications of their work will understand how decisions and policies are made by a coterie of people, some of whom have studied together or find some solace in each other's views of any scientific or medical problem. It is also amazing to find how small a research area often is in terms of numbers of people. Often they have been students of an eminent name.

The family tree is well worth exploring and is certainly true for the ME research field and who holds the reins of decision-making in ME treatments and research.

The All Party Parliamentary Group (APPG) on ME

In 1998, a year after Tony Blair won the General Election, an All Party Parliamentary Group on ME was set up in the UK Parliament by Tony Wright, an MP for Great Yarmouth. He had been persuaded by a local group, BRAME (The Blue Ribbon for the Awareness of ME), to set it up. This organisation had 3 major aims:

1. To create an increased awareness and understanding of ME

2. To help raise funds for research

3. To show support for those affected by ME

They attended inquiries, NICE, the Department of Work and Pensions and the All Party Group. It had 2 main activists, one a patient and the other her mother who was the carer. They harried government departments and local authorities and deserve the accolade of us all. At the first debate in Parliament in 1998 the problems of patients were outlined by several MPs on a non-party basis. In reply the Minister of State said that the current All Party Parliamentary Group has the following purpose:

To improve the lives of people with ME. The APPG will achieve this by working collaboratively to stimulate greater understanding and awareness of the illness, and tackling key policy areas to improve outcomes for people affected by ME. The key areas that the APPG identified for enquiry were as follows:

- The service framework for caring for people with ME
- Funding available for service provision for caring for people with ME
- Estimating numbers of adults and children with ME, those who are severely affected and annual funding required to provide adequate health care services
- Plans for new clinical services where currently none exist

- What happens to people who have secondary referral but no local service exists
- Ways in which patient outcomes are measured and how this compares with patients' perspectives

Other issues that the APPG were to address included diagnostic criteria being used and the level of understanding of both symptoms and impact on patients in primary, secondary and specialist care centres. The APPG also wanted to look at training of health professionals and their understanding of different interventions and management strategies. The aim was to increase the knowledge of ME at all levels of health care and implement appropriate treatment, support and assessment. Organisations and individuals affected by ME were also invited to submit written evidence to the APPG.

In 2009 Dr Des Turner, the MP for Brighton Kemptown, became Chair of the APPG and took up the cudgels on behalf of those with ME by taking on the Chair. He instituted an inquiry entitled 'Inquiry into NHS Service Provision for ME' which was published in March 2010.[54] The inquiry made 11 key recommendations that were flagged up as 'vital and urgent for the long overdue improvement in the Government's support to the 250,000 people with M.E. in the UK and their carers.' (2010: p3). We reproduce below sections of the Inquiry that illustrate how, since the reports of the Government Medical Director, Liam Donaldson in 2002 and the Gibson Inquiry of 2006, many of the problems remained the same as far as patients and carers were concerned despite the earlier recommendations being thorough in how the improvements to services were to be delivered.

- Review of Current Treatments: The main treatments offered to patients were described and surveys carried out

---

[54] Inquiry into NHS Service Provision for ME: Westminster, March 2010

in health centres and online surveys conducted through patient support groups. The total number of patients who were surveyed for the inquiry was over 4,000. The surveys found that pacing is arguably the best current treatment that enables patients to manage their lives to some extent.
- Review of Adult Services: The lack of provision of specialist care was underlined. Poor diagnosis due to lack of training and knowledge meant patients being left with little or no treatment and support. Referrals for specialist care varied considerably across regions. Primary Care Trusts (PCT)s were surveyed for information on provision, 91 out of 133 PCTs failed to even respond to the APPG request for information.
- Review of Children's Services: Many areas only offer services to ME patients over the age of 16 years and therefore children under this age are frequently neglected. This can be due to lack of diagnosis or lack of access to services. Children's needs are more focused on social and educational support in addition to the recognized treatments for adults.
- Training: The inquiry found that doctors receive little or no training for treating ME patients. It may be on their radar but there is no consistency in training. The inquiry stated that "it is essential there is increased training for medical students and junior doctors." (2010: p14). In addition, the NICE guidelines explicitly state that "Every person diagnosed with ME should be offered acceptance and understanding" (2010: p15) which was found to be not the case where practitioners lack the knowledge and training to diagnose and offer appropriate treatment.
- Research: The inquiry urged investment into research into the causes of ME and appropriate treatments. This was at the time of the XMRV trials that linked the virus to ME – later to be discredited. The MRC funding mentioned in the inquiry subsequently went to research grants led by scientists in the field of psychology, most notably the much criticized PACE Trial.
- Benefits: The inquiry stated that "due to the nature of the disease and the lack of knowledge surrounding it, it is very

difficult for those affected to get the support they need" (2010: p17). This is borne out by the account of Kenny's experiences of claiming welfare benefits in the case study at the end of this chapter.

Ironically, the much vaunted XMRV research which the Inquiry hoped would shine a light on the causes of ME resulted in broken careers for some scientists, most notably Dr Judy Mikovits and others at the Whittemore Peterson Research Institute in Nevada was highlighted. However, the XMRV research also brought in new researchers such as Jonas Blomberg from Sweden and Ian Lipkin from USA who were not turned away despite the subsequent negative findings and have continued their involvement in ME. In the inquiry Dr Esther Crawley said in her oral evidence, that she expected "the MRC to have a number of applications for research grants into the field. Dr Crawley pointed out that as more doctors and specialists become interested in the area, there will be more grant applications, thereby increasing the research funding" (2010: p16). Sadly, the truth proved to be the opposite and even the psychiatric explanations apparently resulted in little more research.

There was concern amongst MPs and other politicians about the conduct of the APPG and, in particular, the behaviour of visitors in a parliamentary committee. APPGs grew in increasing numbers after 1997 and there was variation from a group on carers to a group on chocolate. A member of Dr Gibson's staff once said cynically that we could set up a group on beaches, ensuring that we visited many. APPGs are supported by consultancies, large companies as well as by patient groups. Visits and conferences were all funded by these influential organizations who gain the advantage of discussing policies, free passes into the House of Westminster and debates and questions can be held and asked. They can play a strong part in policy formation.

The APPG on ME Review in 2010 recommended the following code of practice.

- The APPG and the Secretariat (Action for ME and The ME Association) accepts the WHO Classification of ME as a neurological condition, recognized by the Dept. of Health as long term.
- The APPG is committed to improve health, social care, education and employment opportunities for those with ME.
- Meetings of the APPG should be held in public and those attending should adhere to best practice in their conduct at meetings.

The APPG also recognized the 2008 Research Expert Group led by Professor Stephen Holgate of Southampton University who was to review current research, identify new research opportunities and encourage understanding of the disease. A section in the 2010 review called on the attendees of the APPG to behave in a manner allowing the committee to complete its work without undue harassment or interruption. Notes on the meeting in 2009 reveal that "the meeting got off to an extremely regrettable start – all due to a very small section of the audience making repeated and sometimes very aggressive interruptions about various administrative matters" [55]. "The APPG and the Secretariat recognize the connection between the behaviour of individuals in meetings and the ability of the APPG to address its business effectively" (2010: p7).

Despite the continuous tensions with some patient support groups before and after the Gibson Inquiry and the one on NHS provision for people with ME the report came out. The hostility continued and this detracted from achieving positive responses from

---

[55] http://tinyurl.com/zx8p2a8

government. Consideration by the MPs to get government to sit up and take notice, despite letters to and discussions with ministers, were accompanied by protests about the importance of patient groups on the APPG before and after their production and there was a strong resistance to any support for a psychiatric approach even if accompanied by the favoured biomedical approach. Discussions of both reports did take place at APPG meetings. A minister, Mike O'Brien, at a meeting of the APPG in 2009 made the following comments:

- The 2002 Chief Medical Officer's (Dr Liam Donaldson) report was a turning point for ME but recommendations to clinical, administrative and funding bodies were unmet

- The APPG Report was a serious and obvious contribution but that meeting the individual needs of patients through appropriate care pathways was complex and the needs were not being met

- Management of ME differs between PCTs (Primary Care Trusts) and service providers remain unclear and/or sceptical about treatments

- ME support groups need to work together at local level for better services

- More hard evidence and biomedical research is needed

- There are problems faced by patients of ME dealing with Dept. of Work and Pensions and the benefit systems

So the Report underlined the various recommendations made by the APPG but, as the Nursing Times[56] pointed out, rather cynically 'APPGs have no power and this will be ignored as was the Gibson

---

[56] The Nursing Times 'Parliamentary Group hits out at lack of support for ME' March, 2010

Report into ME'. The Nursing Times also drew attention to the APPG's comments by Des Turner on the lack of understanding of ME by those in the front line of health care and social security departments, also illustrated by our case study of Kenny at the end of this chapter.

We are particularly concerned by the failure of many primary care trusts to fund any services for ME/CFS patients, especially children and the most severely affected. We are also deeply concerned by the poor knowledge that many doctors have about this illness and by the failure of the DWP and its contractor (ATOS) to understand its adverse impact on many patients' ability to undertake regular work. (APPG final report, 2010).

In the same edition of Nursing Times other medical issues are raised surrounding ME, such as the donation of blood by those suffering from ME and why graded exercise and CBT should be the only treatments given when the condition is defined by WHO as a neurological disease?

A reference to the results of the 2010 APPG report on facilities was drawn in the minutes of a meeting between held in May 2011 between the APPG and the then coalition minister for care services, Paul Burstow. A member of the APPG, Annette Brooke MP, noted that although APPG had recently heard promising news from Professor Stephen Holgate about ME research, little if any improvement in NHS care has occurred for people with ME since the 2010 Inquiry by APPG. The Group raised several points with Paul Burstow, most importantly that although the government say repeatedly that they recognize ME as a neurological condition this belief is not disseminated through the Department of Health or Department for Work and Pensions. Many GPs still do not accept that ME is a neurological condition. Also that there continues to be very little NHS provision for those suffering from severe ME and what does exist is difficult to access due to the disabling nature of ME. It was noted that some people are still being wrongly assessed as having mental health disorders and referred for inappropriate treatment. In addition, the Department for Work and Pensions continually denies ME patients social security benefits related to their incapacity to work due to illness. The APPG also drew attention to safeguarding issues, where parents of children suffering from ME had wrongly been reported to social services as 'negligent'. This whole experience up to 2010 was described to me by Dr Des Turner as a 'waste of time and really when what is needed is so obvious'.

What we need is a Parliamentary debate!

Early in the Blair government (1997-2007) following the birth of the All Party Parliamentary Group on ME, Tony Wright, the MP for Great Yarmouth, pressurized for a debate. It may not have had the same level of support as generated for the debates and committees on the subject of banning fox hunting but it ensured that it was at least on a sub-agenda. It could not replace cancer or mental health as the two government priorities. Debates also turn up interesting points and those on the benches were informed that the APPG group was set up in 1987 in the House of Commons. The MPs all referred to constituents who were incapacitated by ME and the need for biomedical research.

In a non-committal response the Minister, Tessa Jowell, stated that 'individual doctors decide in consultation with their patients'. She went on to acknowledge that this would cause 'problems of inconsistency' and would not give us the evidence to cure the condition. There was a recognition of the problems but she said the Chief Medical Officers report would lead to relief for those who were suffering. It did not do this when it appeared in 2002.

Professional integrity and in-fighting

The recent case of Dr Nigel Speight has come to the attention of those concerned for the well-being of ME patients, particularly children. Dr Speight has a long and illustrious career treating patients with ME, particularly young children. He has been medical advisor to several national ME charities. He also appeared as an expert speaker on treatments for ME on the BBC Panorama programme in 1999 'Sick and Tired' which questioned the validity of the psychological approach to treatment endorsed by the NHS. The background to his case cannot be ignored – he has consistently opposed the views of high-level government policy makers. He was a major contributor to the film Voices from the Shadows, the story of five ME patients and their carers and also featuring Professor Leonard Jason and Professor Malcolm Hooper. He also gave the pre-conference dinner speech at the IIMEC10 conference in London with some horrific details of the cases of severely affected children who were removed from the families. In his 2012 handout following the film, Dr Speight explained how the official understanding of ME was misguided, following on from a research paper written in 1972 by two psychiatrists who suggested that the outbreak of 1955 at the Royal Free Hospital in London was due to mass hysteria among the mainly female nurses and doctors. The two scientists did not actually see any patients but simply looked a case records from the time.

This paper was the start of the process whereby the medical profession retreated into a position of disbelief regarding ME, and allowed the area to be taken over by psychiatry for about 30 years. For a while things seemed about to improve with the publication of the CMO report in 2002 which concluded that "ME is a genuine illness and patients should be not be dismissed as malingerers". Unfortunately this did not last and the subsequent publication of the NICE Guidelines (with their emphasis on the value of CBT) has led to something of a comeback for the psychiatric viewpoint.[57]

As a result of his voicing concerns about the direction of treatment and research for ME (and for treating children with ME as having an organic illness), Dr Speight's integrity came under the spotlight, after a complaint was made to the General Medical Council (GMC). He was called to attend a hearing in front of the GMC during April 2016 which resulted in him being suspended from any activity concerning ME. This is an extract from his public statement of 22 April 2016:

> [The GMC] have imposed interim conditions on my registration mirroring the voluntary restrictions I had offered for a period of 15 months. The conditions prevent me from carrying out any work in relation to ME in either a paid or unpaid capacity......Please also understand that these restrictions even extend to preventing me speaking or lecturing on the subject of ME. To my fellow members of the authoring committee of the International Consensus report on paediatric ME/CFS, I am afraid I also have to withdraw from future contributions.[58]

We spoke to Nigel Speight recently and below are some of the cases he has represented. Over the past thirty years Nigel Speight has been involved with over forty cases of child protection proceedings in the UK against families of children with ME. Proceedings were driven by a variety of agencies against families – pediatricians, child psychiatrists, educational authorities, former spouses and social workers. The courts did not uphold the accusations of neglect or abuse in any of these cases. The controversy between the psychological and biological view of the

---

[57] http://voicesfromtheshadowsfilm.co.uk/nigel-speight-me-handout/
[58] http://www.investinme.org/Documents/GMC/Speight%20Letter%20GMC%2022-4-2016.pdf

illness played a significant role in the reported cases where the failure to make a correct diagnosis was responsible for the involvement of outside agencies such as social service departments. Dr Speight was particularly active in representing families of children with ME during the period 1985-2015 in his role as a pediatrician with a special interest in the illness and acting on behalf of families at the request of ME charities (AYME, TYMES TRUST). Occasionally he was approached directly by the families to represent them in legal proceedings.

The types of scenario described by Dr Speight are of three main types. In one example the threat to separate a child from her parents involved the misdiagnosis of ME as Munchausen Syndrome by Proxy whereby symptoms were seen as psychological responses to a dysfunctional family relationship. This case saw the child put on a register for 'Emotional Abuse' and plans were made to start care proceedings to remove the child into foster care. Dr Speight's intervention corrected the diagnosis to that of ME and thus the decision to remove the child from its parents was reversed.

Another scenario described by Dr Speight was the forced treatment of a child with a multi-disciplinary therapeutic regime, CBT (Cognitive Behavioural Therapy) and GET (Graded Exercise Therapy). In this case the child was subjected to forced physical activity, against the wishes of both parents and child. The resulting state of health was a rapid physical deterioration. Clashes between the parents and medical professionals fuelled the case against the parents. The child was made Ward of Court and only when it became evident that the treatment regime was having a negative effect did the Court accept they had been misled.

We find that among both medical professionals and the general public, there is a disbelief in the illness known as ME. This can cause a family member or friend to report a parent to social services for emotional abuse or neglect. Dr Speight found that this is particularly hard to refute when the family member or friend is a teacher, nurse or other professional. Pediatricians, social workers and the judiciary can add enormous amounts of stress to a family and child through false accusations. With ME the stress can trigger further decline and delay in recovery.

When we investigated the events leading up to Dr Speight's suspension we found secrecy around the divulgence of the names of the original complainants and the interests of committee members. Suffice it to say that we know that there are correlations with alternative views of how to treat children and the basis for these. In particular, in one case the abandonment of Dr Speight's treatments had sadly led to a worsening of the ME, it is alleged. The whole history of the events leading to his suspension has been investigated. Principally it would seem to have resulted from the biomedical/ psychiatric divide with the latter in the ascendancy of control. In October 2016 we were pleased to learn that the General Medical Council withdrew the limitations it had imposed on Dr Nigel Speight's ability to practice and restored his licence in full with no constraints. These restrictions to Dr Speight's professional freedoms should never have been imposed upon him by the GMC in the first place.

The minefield of ME is no doubt a deterrent for many looking for a career in treatment and research. Dr Speight's suspension from any type of work relating to ME went against the wishes of those organizations devoted to supporting patients and finding alternative treatments to the psychological approach. How can the background to this case, where professional rivalries and opposing views on ME would seem to cast their murky shadow, be justified in the interests of those suffering from ME? No doubt cases like that of Dr Speight will continue to be challenged on many fronts, and no doubt disagreements over treatments will continue and thus progress be thwarted.

Trying to insure when diagnosed with ME

The Gibson Inquiry addressed the problem of individuals and their success at obtaining insurance cover for ME and absence from work or disability allowance. This is shown in the inquiry report as an answer to a parliamentary question from P. Duncan in 2002.

Mr. Peter Duncan: To ask the Secretary of State for Work and Pensions whether a claim for Disability Living Allowance in respect of ME may be classified as relating to mental illness. [87128]

Maria Eagle: Entitlement to Disability Living Allowance depends on the effects that severe physical or mental disability has on a person's need for personal care and/or their ability to walk, and not on particular disabilities or diagnoses. The benefit is available to people with myalgic encephalomyelitis (which can have a physical basis or a psychological basis, or can be due to a combination of factors) on exactly the same terms as other severely disabled people, and they can qualify for it provided that they meet the usual entitlement conditions.

There are staff members at the medical assessment centres who dismiss claims as irrelevant, trivial and attention seeking. Few can pass the first hurdle and from first-hand knowledge we have heard one medical assessor dismiss the claims of patients as 'mere frippery'. Advisors to the Department of Work and Pensions have been awarded consultancies with medical insurance companies e.g.

UNUM Provident. Some of the names already predominant in the ME field have appeared in other parts of the world of ME, e.g. grant award committees in the field of science. Whilst difficult to ensure the impartiality of a medical professor steeped in camaraderie and back scratching, the problem requires addressing. As reports of old pals are exposed in business, universities, clubs etc. then the time is ripe for a full analysis of the individuals concerned.

ME and social security benefits

It has come to our attention that many sufferers of ME have faced a long struggle to find some financial support during their illness. In the UK those with long term illnesses are eligible for social security benefits after assessment by health professionals. A major change in financial support for the long term ill came about in 2008 when the former Work and Pensions Secretary in the Conservative government, Iain Duncan-Smith, replaced Incapacity Benefit, 'a social security benefit payable to those who are incapable of work because of illness or disability', with the controversial Employment and Support Allowance:

Employment and Support Allowance (ESA) is a new way of helping people with an illness or disability to move into work, if they are able.

ESA offers personalised support and financial help, so that recipients can engage in appropriate work, if they are able. It provides access to a specially trained personal adviser and a wide range of further services including employment, training and condition management support, to help recipients manage and cope with their illness or disability in a work context. Central to ESA is the new medical assessment called the Work Capability Assessment which assesses what a person can rather than can't do and identifies the health related support that might be needed. Most people claiming ESA will be expected to take appropriate steps to help prepare for work, including attending a series of work-focused interviews with their personal adviser. Under ESA, if a recipient has an illness or disability that severely affects their ability to work, they will get increased financial support and will not be expected to prepare for a return to work; however, they can volunteer to do so if they want to.

The new benefit rules have impacted on many people with long-term illnesses and particularly those with ME. Duncan-Smith stated that the new benefit aimed to encourage more sick and disabled people into work. There are currently 2.3 million people who are classified as unable to work due to disability or illness. The other social security benefit that would be appropriate for those with severe cases of ME is the Personal Independence Payment (PIP) replacing the Disability Living Allowance.

Personal Independence Payment (PIP)

To be eligible you must have a long-term health condition or disability and face difficulties with 'daily living' or getting around. You must have had these difficulties for 3 months and expect them to last for at least 9 months, unless you're terminally ill (you don't expect to live more than 6 months).

Daily living difficulties

You may get the daily living component of PIP if you need help with things like:

- preparing or eating food
- washing, bathing and using the toilet

- dressing and undressing
- reading and communicating
- managing your medicines or treatments
- making decisions about money
- engaging with other people

Mobility difficulties

You may get the mobility component of PIP if you need help going out or moving around.

How you are assessed

Your claim will be assessed by an independent healthcare professional to help DWP work out the level of help you need. This may be a face-to-face consultation - you'll get a letter explaining why and where you must go. You'll be given a score based on how much help you need. The more help you need, the higher the score you'll get. DWP makes the decision about your claim based on the results of the assessment, application and any supporting evidence you include.[59]

The introduction of the Personal Independence Payment caused a major controversy in the 2016 Budget. The former Chancellor, George Osborne, proposed to change the assessment criteria for PIPs to cut the amount payable to claimants thereby saving the government £1.3 billion a year. He was forced to abandon the cuts due to cross party opposition and the dramatic resignation of Duncan-Smith.

The Labour Party leader, Jeremy Corbyn, applauded his resignation and the U-turn in policy but more importantly called

---

[59] www.gov.uk/hmrc

for "an examination of the appalling way in which people with disabilities go through these availability-for-work tests."[60]

Interestingly, the first question at the 2016 conference in London (see Annex 1) between the scientists and patients was concerned with 'getting insurance'.

Professor Tom Shakespeare, University of East Anglia, and Ian have raised along with many others how an approach to benefit awards are underpinned by a hypothesis or theory,[61] or 'allegedly' underpinned. The hypothesis and how it is used in the process of benefit delivery and in assessment of conditions like ME was discussed in the Chapter 1. The government has several projects under which it delivers benefits e.g. Work Capability Assessment (WCA), which along with Incapacity Benefit, Job Seekers Allowance etc. have seen many young people on such payments. Attempts to hide the true jobless numbers have seen some figures not included in such statistics. Assessment and eligibility were affected by Personal Capacity Assessment in the mid-90s. The Labour Government of 1997-2010 saw the introduction of 'Pathway to Work' politics in the mid-2000s followed by the Employment Support Allowance (ESP) in 2008. There were 4 policy changes at this time:

1. The introduction of a more stringent Work Capability Assessment (WCA) to replace the Personal Capacity Assessment (PCA) at three months rather than six months into the claim. The WCA uses a points-based system and examines what activities the claimant is capable of undertaking. All former Incapacity Benefit claimants have had to be retested for ESA.

---

[60] http://www.telegraph.co.uk/news/politics/conservative/12198625 (Sunday 27 March 2016)

[61] Waddell G. and Aylward M. (2005) *Models of Sickness and Disability applied to common health problems*. Centre for Psychosocial and Disability Research, School of Medicine, University of Cardiff.

2. The expectation that most of those on ESA will be fit to return to work and the establishment of a Work-Related Activity component (WRAG), on which people are expected to take part in training courses or similar activities aimed at promoting their readiness to work.

3. Introduction of sanctions against those who fail to comply with work-related activities.

4. The establishment of a Support Group comprising those who are not expected to return to work and who are exempt from work-related activities. This group also receives an additional premium on top of their ESA, thus ostensibly addressing socio-economic disadvantages." [62]

Further changes since 2012 have been described by Shakespeare in his paper (2016). The gradual shift over these years as seen fewer on benefits like ESA and an increase in those available and ready to work. The move was meant to focus on the effects of the disabling condition and not the condition itself.

Applicants must first go through a 13 week 'assessment phase'. There are two separate assessments:

- *limited capability for work assessment* measures a person's ability to perform certain activities relating to physical, mental, cognitive and intellectual function and determines whether the individual qualifies for ESA;
- *limited capability for work-related activity assessment* determines the rate of ESA that will be paid after the first 13 weeks and whether the claimant will be required to undertake any work-related activity as a condition of entitlement." (ibid, 2016)

---

[62] Shakespeare, Tom, Watson N. and Alghaib O.A. (2016) 'Blaming the victim, all over again: Waddell and Aylwards biophyschosocial (BPS) model of disability" in *Critical Social Policy 2016*, Vol 36(4): 1-20

Some were still assessed as unable to work or with limited ability and appear in the Support Group. The ESA in the Work-Related Activity Group (WRAG) had a 1-year limit. Others may be moved to Jobseekers Allowance (JSA) which is means-tested after 6 months and is lower than ESA. WCA has been tackled by support groups and in particular the ATOS, the French health insurance contractor which won the administration contract after a competitive process and has now been replaced by Maximus, an American for-profit company. We should note that the change from Incapacity Benefit to Employment Support Allowance and from Personal Capacity Assessment to Work Capability Assessment was a policy change too far. The companies used healthcare professionals and were in league with the Department for Work and Pensions. A hard edge assessment was needed and not the gentle approval of 'community' General Practitioners. There was little assessed of any psychosocial effects on capabilities for work. There is a common reluctance in many quarters for allowing the re-entry of someone who has been 'a problem' back into the work force.

There is little evidence to indicate that any of these policies address the individual's problems including access to work. Patchy successes may have been recorded but they are not universal. Let us look at some of the experiences of those we spoke to. The following is a description of events provided by Peter.

Case Study: Peter

Peter was diagnosed with ME/CFS in 2005. The diagnosis was accepted and undisputed by his employer, a major multinational financial services firm, and has remained unchallenged by GPs and consultants since that time. Peter held medical insurance through an international provider of life insurance, pensions and asset management. This company appointed an independent medical examiner who claimed that Peter suffered from USO – Undifferentiated Somatoform Disorder – which is the term given to a person with physical complaints lasting over 6 months and which cannot be attributed to a known medical condition.

The insurance company continued to challenge the original diagnosis by GPs and consultants in the UK and terminated Peter's claim for medical insurance on the incorrect classification of his illness by the insurance company's staff as a mental and behavioural disorder. This, of course, was in contradiction to the WHO classification under code ICD-10 and indeed that of the UK Chief Medical Officer in 2002 who stated that the Dept. of Health recognises ME/CFS as a genuine and disabling neurological disorder.

Peter decided to make a legal challenge to the insurance company's decision and carried out research into their methods and process of both definition and diagnosis. He discovered a chain of shabby research and decision making mechanisms based on one-sided medical literature used to substantiate the diagnosis and the involvement of the company's two medical consultants, who happened to be psychiatrists, rather than biomedical practitioners. The insurance company had built a flawed case based on the perception of the disease from a purely psychological argument and ignored the wider and international definitions and diagnosis of ME/CFS which the WHO classification illustrates. Peter was convinced that the employment of psychiatrists by the insurance company, as independent medical advisers, proved that there was an "imbalance in power between the parties and their vested interests and collusion with the insurance company" (Letter from Peter to his legal representatives).

Peter believes "that there is a serious issue with disability insurance such as income protection benefit. This is obviously because of ill-health and vulnerability of the claimants at that point in time of the claim and that rogue insurers have exploited the situation. This is especially the case with ME due to the severity of the disability itself." (*ibid*). His appeal against the decision of the insurance company is ongoing and the hope is that the vast amount of scientific and legal evidence he has produced in support of his case will finally win the day.

As we argue in our last chapter, there is a hypothesis now published which questions not the details of the benefit systems but the underlying model paramount in Establishment circles that pervades our definition of disability. It is our contention that this relates to the history of the definition of ME. The latter may have more complex explanations of causes in contrast to the one-event gives one-problem approach. Another example is that of Kenny which we outline below.

Case Study: Kenny

This is the story of Kenny, narrated by himself, who fought for benefits, was awarded then declined, threatened and reinstated. He was, throughout his ordeal, dealt with by the bureaucracy of the UK government in an unpredictable and irrational manner.

> Prior to the onset of severe ill health, I had what might be called 'fulminating' or background Crohn's Disease - it rumbled away and occasionally flared up, but was never actually recognised, and rarely if ever had any appreciable effect on my activities. I also had gradually deteriorating Seasonal Affective Disorder; every winter from the age of about 12, I would have a bout of depression sometime in winter, which as time went on became longer and deeper and involved more physical symptoms. All that sounds dire, but actually, I spent all my spare time backpacking, hill walking,

cycling and cross-country skiing; I was an absolute endorphin addict! I would not walk if I could run...my job involved running up and down countless flights of stairs in a day, and I never thought twice about it.

In 1988, the year that everything fell apart, I first of all spent a week in hospital following a mistaken diagnosis of a particularly virulent cancer, then spent several months limping about due to a knee injury, and finally went down with what was diagnosed as double viral pneumonia. It was after this that I found my health had completely changed, and very much for the worse; first of all, I suffered severe, suicidal depression that simply did not go away in springtime, then I began to suffer stomach problems and lost weight, and suffered bouts of virtually instantaneous crippling fatigue that were utterly unpredictable and varied in type. All these things left me unable to work; I lost my job and went on benefits.

I was diagnosed as having Post-Viral Fatigue Syndrome quite rapidly, certainly within a year; but to this day, I do not think I have ever been treated specifically for this, I have certainly never attended or even been informed of the existence of any clinic that treats chronic fatigue. Initially I was treated as suffering from depression; when my stomach problems continued that was eventually investigated as being not related and diagnosed as IBS [Irritable Bowel Syndrome], which was then treated as Crohn's disease, and somewhere along the way my official diagnosis became "IBD/Crohn's?" with a statement in my medical notes that I suffered from Chronic Fatigue Syndrome.

Mostly, my treatments have been ad hoc courses of antidepressants or steroids, as a reaction to severe bouts of stomach problems or depression. Fatigue itself, despite its accompanying cognitive problems and catastrophic effects on my entire lifestyle, economically and socially, was simply not treated; rather more I think, seen as just another symptom, very sad but what to do...

Did you seek help or assistance from anyone in public life e.g. politicians?

It never even occurred to me, until I started having problems with the benefits system. Prior to that, I was unaware of any mismatch between the reality of my ill health, and the perception of it in political circles. First of all, I went onto Statutory Sick Pay - no problems there. Then I went onto Incapacity Benefit - no problems there to begin with, the doctor saw me, and signed me off as unfit to work, every so often. He did have a fairly good idea of what I was struggling with, I would tell him about my voluntary activities and how able to do them, plus of course the times I was totally incapacitated.

Eventually my National Insurance payments ran out, and I went onto Income Support. My assessments under IB [Invalidity Benefit], and then IS [Income Support], were always late, and to be honest I found them rather bizarre. I never knew what kind of assessor I'd get; sometimes it would seem perfunctory, on another occasion the assessor seemed very clued up and actually told me I was entitled to an "Ill health" top-up to my benefits. Subsequent to that assessment, my benefits went up without my even applying for the top up, no doubt as a result of this doctor's intervention. It made a big difference to my health, it was something like £20 a week so it paid for the gluten-free food that was really expensive and hard to find then.

In about 1997, when I fell ill again after a period of employment, I was put onto ESA [Employment and Support Allowance]. That, from the very beginning, was not a good experience, even under Labour. There was a WCA [Work Capability Assessment] where I seem to remember getting 9 points out of the 15 needed to qualify as sick; I can't remember, but I think it was the one where the assessor said to me as I left that I would definitely qualify, I had scored the 15. I was very annoyed at him lying brazenly to me like that; it was only years afterwards that I discovered the DWP decision makers were being overruled and points downgraded by their bosses, which was actually illegal as they had not been present at the WCA. I, feeling like my limbs were made of lead some days, was aghast and of course appealed against the decision, and the official reaction was telling.

I remember reading the letter I was sent by the DWP (or whatever they called themselves at the time) with the information on how to appeal. What it said, in essence, was that if I appealed, I would be on half rate benefits (£45 p/week) for an indeterminate length of time while the appeal was processed. If the appeal failed, I would be liable to prosecution for fraud. If on the other hand I was willing to admit I was fit to work and sign on as unemployed, then I would get more money than this, straight away. This latter carrot was mentioned twice. It was breath-taking in its cynicism. You could see that the assumption was that people claiming to be ill were actually just after as much money as they could get, and this letter was designed to tempt them to sign on as unemployed instead. Alternatively - or perhaps in light of later events, I should say, also - the people who designed this system really didn't care about people who really were ill. They didn't accept that the system's findings could ever be wrong, and if the assessments were wrong, well, frightening seriously ill people just didn't matter, they didn't care what harm this did. When I realised this, I felt a chill, and thought, "There is real malice behind this." I have never forgotten that moment; it was a paradigm shift in my thinking, a mental iceberg turning over and showing me hidden truths. I won the appeal at Tribunal, as I have done all my appeals, but for something like nine months I basically just stayed in bed, too stressed, ill and broke to be doing anything else.

The WCA paperwork that I received when appealing really opened my eyes to the fact that things were not normal at WCA's; at one I was asked how I was as I came in the door, and taking it as a mere social greeting I murmured, "Fine, fine" which was my usual greeting no matter how bad I was. Saying that really counted against me when it came to points.

In other instances, outright lies were told, that flatly contradicted what I had said, or were distortions of the truth that turned black to white by omitting context.

As a result of these experiences, I became very determined that I would have future WCA's recorded. By now, I was doing much research online about the process and various claimants' experiences, and knew of the potential pitfalls when dealing with ATOS [which] I found to be a bureaucratic Cerberus: one face nice and very competent (the front office staff, and on occasion the assessors), the other (hidden) side utterly untrustworthy and as truthful as a crack addict asking for a loan.

For one WCA in 2012 I asked for a recorded assessment, which was agreed to and arranged for an appointed time. I turned up with a friend as witness, because I knew that there was a hidden extra that had been inserted into the ATOS paperwork. The Data Protection Act requires that all parties being recorded give their permission, and permit the data to be held by the controller of the data, in this case I think the DWP. Fair enough. However, ATOS had also inserted a clause, which needed to be signed, in which the claimant stated that they would not take any legal action against ATOS. This was not legally required by the Data Protection Act, and it was something which I was not willing to do - by now, I was less than happy with the assessment process. Having been severely impacted health-wise by previous assessments, I wanted myself, or if necessary my next of kin, to be able to sue ATOS for criminal negligence or corporate manslaughter. I was not willing to enter into a separate contract with ATOS, giving up my legal rights.

So I refused to sign that section. I signed the rest, as required by law, but scored out the extra section indemnifying ATOS. It was all very amicable; the front office staff didn't make the system, I had no grievance against them (quite the opposite, I thought they did a great job under terrible conditions) and they were very matter of fact. Phone calls were made and returned, and I was told that I would not be assessed if the form was not signed in its entirety, and that I would be put down as a DNA (Did Not Attend) - which would normally lead to an immediate cessation of benefits. At this point, with a witness, I stated that I was willing to be assessed, willing to meet the legal requirements of the DWP for being assessed, but unwilling to forgo my right to take legal action. I was told again I could not be assessed, and I left. My immediate action thereafter was to phone the DWP and tell them what had occurred, so that any Did Not Attend that arrived would be ignored; I spoke to a very sympathetic low level DWP worker who put the information in my file, and told me that my benefits would continue.

Future DWP workers were not so low level, and not so sympathetic. I received a somewhat agitated phone call from the DWP within days; why was I unwilling to sign, would I agree to sign if another WCA was arranged? I reiterated my stance. The employee said they were very keen to sort this out before my benefits stopped, could they phone me back tomorrow? The next day, I was scheduled to be in hospital having a colonoscopy; under general anaesthetic in the morning, and recovering for the afternoon, so having said this I suggested the day after that and we agreed this would be done. The next day, upon coming out of the operating theatre, lo and behold, I had missed calls from Livingston - the DWP. Still high as a kite on opiates, and with dire warnings not to make important decisions or operate machinery ringing in my ears, I was released to go home, and once more, the DWP rang. A female Team Leader took over the call from a subordinate. She told me that I MUST sign that section of the form. I could not be assessed without it. My benefits would stop, and I would have no more benefits of any sort until such times as I signed. She was exceptionally clear on that point; there was no ambiguity possible. I was given a stern warning that signing this was a DWP requirement and my money would stop: "Well, then, I'm afraid we are at an impasse, because I will not do it." And we hung up.

My money continued as before; it took a further year for my Work Capability Assessment to be rearranged. When I arrived, they had removed the extra clause from the form, and for the first time ever, I scored 15 points without needing to appeal. It's now 51 months since that award, and in fear and anger, I once more await the dreaded ESA50 form to drop on my doormat, as the WCA system falls apart. Now that ATOS have left the contract, I wonder how their successors Maximus will do?"

Our thanks to Kenny for sharing his experience with us. The reader may well be confused by the processes and procedures of assessment. It is hard to imagine how anyone with a chronic, incapacitating illness like ME can cope with these hurdles.

Fortunately, there are some high profile campaigners fighting the injustices portrayed in this book. One example is the British film director, Ken Loach, has been awarded a second Palme d"Or at Cannes with his major feature film 'I, Daniel Blake' (2016). The film takes a scathing look at the Department for Work and Pensions assessment process for those with long-term disabilities. The film shocks and challenges the establishment. It portrays the outrage of a victim of the politically motivated social security framework designed with such complexity and inhumanity as to disinherit citizens of their rights. We wonder if the new administration under PM Theresa May will have the courage to put right the mistakes of her predecessors in her quest to create a Britain 'that works for all'?

Chapter 5 – The Biopsychosocial Model

Throughout the preparation of this book we have often wondered why ME has raised such controversy, by whom and on whose behalf. In the last few months of our writing a clue started to emerge. The question has often come up for many years about the role of insurance companies and medical groups who insure for sickness. We have given an account of some personal experiences in those we interviewed and there were many, many more accounts available to us in writing this book. The assessment procedure by both the Department for Work and Pensions and insurance companies denies people the chance of developing a full life. The record shows how prominent individuals, usually psychiatrists, have been employed as consultants to give a psychiatric explanation for ME, thereby changing an individual's right to financial or medical support.

Let us look first at the hypotheses or theory that the experts would underline. It stems from the Biopsychosocial Model of Health (BPS) developed by Dr Gordon Waddell, an orthopaedic surgeon, and Dr Mansel Aylward, a former Chief Medical Officer for Work and Pensions. Their model is based loosely on one of mental distress and attempts to take a multi-factorial approach to assessing disability. It was an approach to the rationalisation of benefit payments that we will outline later in this chapter.

The belief was that it was negative attitudes of e.g. ESA recipients (Employment Support Allowance) for work and not health that led to these health and social problems. This also applied to Work Capability Assessments (WCA) despite many appeals being upheld at Personal Independence Payments in 2012 led to a minister saying "Sickness and disability are best overcome by an appropriate combination of healthcare, rehabilitation, personal effort and social/work adjustments". He went on to say there was a coherent theory behind the assessments, which <u>there was not</u>.

Let us look in a little more detail at this Waddell-Aylward biopsychosocial model. The work was developed in a centre sponsored by Unum insurance. The model was a vague interaction of biological, psychological and social factors and certainly not defined in a precise, evidence-based 'theory'. It is a subject in need of biological factors or units. We will take time to explain the difference between general illness and a disease.

Physical disorders, distress and illness vaguely portend disability. The favourite treatment that stemmed from this approach was for graduated exercise plans and psychological techniques to substitute for say, a surgical treatment. If it were for back pain, an extremely common problem, then 'return to work' is recommended as the perspective. As various disabilities occur the Waddell-Aylward BPS in essence gives advice to return to work with no benefits, but take time off for perhaps a treatment or surgical procedure. Real claimants are supported in opposition to fake beneficiaries.

This is the basis of welfare reform and sickness benefit and therefore serves the interests of insurance companies. It is also a view that interests certain parts of the media – skivers must be sought out. A similar language is used for those with ME. Such language becomes crucial in the arguments over benefit rights and result in bringing psychological factors into the 'illness' discussion. Medical and social are interwoven to dilute the importance of biomedical explanations. Victim blaming is much preferable when you can use it to win an argument.

Medical evidence from chosen practitioners was originally viewed suspiciously but ruses like 'He can walk to the newsagents' or 'He can take his grandchild for a walk' gave medically trained

GPs or consultants the opportunity to dismiss a claim. They were well paid to provide such decisions and as an MP Ian noted how certain doctors were guaranteed to reach a negative assessment whilst others would be more circumspect before reaching a conclusive response to such questions.

In their paper, Shakespeare et al [63], point out several important inconsistencies and there is no resolution from evidence. It is another example of policy coming before evidence, and there are many other examples given. The critique of this paper certainly does not justify the Waddell-Aylward model and it may be much more complicated given that scientific technologies are now beginning to bear fruit.

However, disabled people, including those with ME, cannot foresee great improvements in benefits or better facilities in the job market to suit their talents. Whilst it is true that health conditions can affect one's mental functioning going back to the same job is not the answer. Employers should be 'encouraged, supported and regulated' and people taken on with full support into the workplace.

Conclusion

As we watch the politicians, read our medical literature, watch the research developments, student training, efforts of charities etc. to take on serious and important issues, we have angry thoughts.

Where do the resources come from when we use what we have for apparent 'vanity' projects like high speed trains to and from London - projects that the media generally shame the government

---

[63] Shakespeare, Tom, Watson N. and Alghaib O.A. (2016) 'Blaming the victim, all over again: Waddell and Aylwards biophyschosocial (BPS) model of disability" in *Critical Social Policy 2016*, Vol 36(4): 1-20

into providing, and on and on it goes. We convince our leaders and our representatives in local and national government into prioritising this or that.

If a most eminent celebrity or royal personage had ME we bet it would all change!

Chapter 6 - The Future, not the Past

Stephen Holgate Professor of Immuno-pharmacology at the University of Southampton, was Chair of the CMRC (CFS/ME Research Collaborative) meeting in London in 2013. He welcomed the joining together of forces that would bring about a step change in the amount and quality of research and consultation into chronic fatigue syndrome and ME. Many charities attended the event - Action for ME, Association of-Young People with ME, the Chronic Fatigue Syndrome Research Foundation, the ME Association and ME Research UK. Major research funders like the Medical Research Council (MRC), the National Institute for Health Research (NIHR) and the Wellcome Trust were also present.

Charities such as Invest in ME Research, Tymes Trust and the 25% Group for the severely affected chose not join this group for interesting reasons.

Holgate once addressed the Forward ME group in the House of Lords. He proposed ME might cover 15 different diseases. He admitted that breast cancer, too, can have 14 different types, albeit it looks like a uniform illness. In 2011 he had said there might not be one cause of ME and proposed that the time was ripe to apply many of the new biological technologies e.g. molecular methods. A multidisciplinary approach could look at phenotypes, genotypes, gene expression, cytokines etc. His approach certainly would seem to be more positive than blaming the patient for their over-reaction and hysteria. So had Holgate actually made a start by stating at the time that he was "prepared to listen and take on difficult challenges and continue even if prevailing opinion was against me"?

Actions speak louder than words.

It is illustrative of the situation that nothing has changed with the MRC's policy toward ME – and nothing of note has occurred under Holgate's supervision of the MRC research policy toward ME since he was involved from 2008, other than platitudes.

This is one reason why charity Invest in ME Research refused to join this collaborative – feeling partly also that it was dominated by those who still put forward a biopsychosocial view of ME and still seemingly carrying influence with MRC decision makers.[64]

The charity also objected to a charter, written and agreed by the Collaborative committee and charities taking part, which prevented members from criticising others in the collaborative, for example those who consistently maintained the biopsychosocial view of ME.

They maybe had a point.

The history of MRC spending between 2004-2011 on biomedical research into the aetiology of ME was 0% which contrasted sharply with many other illnesses where vast sums of money were awarded to researchers from government and charity funders. Money, however, was put into psychosocial therapies whilst aetiological studies to prove the physiological nature of the illness received little support. The failure of the PACE trial has further soured the view of those advocating the need for a national policy on the biomedical and biological issues involved in the evaluation of ME. The MRC "Expert Panels" began in 2003. It is now 2016 – 13 years have gone by and the MRC have implemented nothing of any value to either treat or look for causes of ME. Since 2013 there

---

[64] http://www.investinme.org/IIME-Newslet-1304-01.shtml

has been little of note from the MRC that can really be seen to be treating this disease properly. This underlines how ineffectual the MRC attitude and policies and "expert" panels have been toward ME in the last decade.

UK Charity Invest in ME Research recently wrote to the CEO of the MRC, Sir John Savill, requesting that those influencing MRC policies on ME over the last decade should be replaced, that the public funding for the PACE Trial should be requested to be returned to fund other (biomedical) research, and that an inquiry should be held into the PACE trial and MRC policies since the 2002 CMO report [65] [66]

In the UK this disease, which is incurable, has had inadequate therapies, indifferent government attitudes, social stigma and no strong public voice.

There are many pieces of research from across the world looking at neuro-inflammation of the brain, eye dysfunction and the current emphasis is on the immune system in ME patients where various immunological cells vary in their type and numbers as the illness progresses. Other areas of research into dementia, stroke, Asperger's etc. over many years involving biomedical understanding could lead to a confluence of treatment, care and support. Testing by clinical trials of potential drugs or new technologies can give us surprises as with rituximab which was a cancer drug but has a possible future in treatment of ME if trials prove positive. The determination put into treating AIDS, Ebola or Zika is not just because they are viruses but because, like ME, they destroy lives and dreams.

Campaign for success

---

[65] http://investinme.org/newslett-Sep16-01-a.htm
[66] http://www.investinme.org/IIME-Newslet-1511-01.shtml

As we write the controlling government party in the UK is reeling from a battle over the restriction of benefits for the poorer segment of UK society to be balanced against the positive tax benefits for the wealthy. Not an unknown scene in other countries, e.g. the USA. The continual propaganda since the 1970s in the UK is about the advantages of deregulating markets. The anger is growing and it is witnessed too in areas of health like ME where those who run the health service consist of an increasing number of businessmen on the governing boards and chosen general practitioners on commissioning groups, who decide the priorities of illnesses to be treated.

Government after government, party after party have failed to listen and continue to re-organise the NHS in the UK woefully in the direction of privatisation of government control. They have attacked doctors, nurses, social workers and argue about who is and is not an 'entrepreneur' (their term).

In such a system how could a disease like ME be treated seriously when it is claimed that the symptoms are the fault of the individual or are being fabricated?

Politicians, as the playwright David Hare says, 'have become little more than go-betweeners, their principal function is to hand over taxpayers' assets, always in 'car boot sales' and always at way less than market value'.

Many now believe that the movement to change will only come from below, so do we. Hare, again, says

Like Blair before him, Cameron has reduced the act of government to a sort of murmuring grudge, a resentment, in which politicians continually tell the surly people that we lack the necessary virtues for survival in the modern world. They know perfectly well that we hate them, and so their only response is to hate us back. Politics has been reduced to a sort of institutionalised nagging, in which a rack of pampered professionals, cut from the eye of the ruling class, tells everyone else that they don't "get it", and that they must "measure up" and "change their ways". Having discharged their analysis, the preachers then invariably scoot off through wide-open doors to 40th-floor boardrooms to make themselves frictionless fortunes as greasers and lobbyists – or, as they prefer to say, "consultants". [67]

In such a climate we cannot expect much support from our electoral representatives or even medical experts.

Yet even here it is possible for change to occur and for those who retain a sense of morality to question the status quo. At the time of writing some probing questions were being asked in parliament by a Labour MP concerned at the conduct of the those involved in the PACE Trial and the policies of the MRC. Kelvin Hopkins posed questions to the relevant ministers – putting questions that every ME patient or carer would want to ask [68]

Question: 54353   Asked on: 22 November 2016

Department for Business, Energy and Industrial Strategy

Chronic Fatigue Syndrome: Research

To ask the Secretary of State for Business, Energy and Industrial Strategy, if he will take steps to identify those responsible for the Medical Research Council's policies towards ME research over the last decade; and if he will seek those people's removal from positions of influence over future of ME research.

---

[67] Hare, David. *Why the Tory Project is Bust.* The Guardian, Tuesday 8 March 2016.
[68] http://tinyurl.com/h3rnngq

Answer: Answered by: Joseph Johnson 30 November 2016

Management of individual staff within the Medical Research Council is a matter for the MRC as the legal employer.

Question: 54354 Asked on: 22 November 2016

Department for Business, Energy and Industrial Strategy Chronic Fatigue Syndrome

To ask the Secretary of State for Business, Energy and Industrial Strategy, if he will review the policy of the Medical Research Council (MRC) in so far as it relates to addressing the dissatisfaction of ME patients with MRC's approach in this area.

Answer: Answered by: Joseph Johnson 30 November 2016:

The MRC welcomes applications to support research into any aspect of human health and these are subject to peer review and judged in open competition. Awards are made on the basis of the scientific quality of the proposals made. The MRC has promoted research into Chronic Fatigue Syndrome/Myalgic Encephalopathy (CFS/ME) through highlight notices for a number of years.

Concerning dissatisfaction of patients, I will write to the Chair of the Medical Research Council to request an account of the development of relevant policies and in particular how CFS/ME patients' views have been considered. I will deposit a copy of his reply in the Libraries of the House.

Question: 54269 Asked on: 22 November 2016

Department for Business, Energy and Industrial Strategy

Chronic Fatigue Syndrome: Research

To ask the Secretary of State for Business, Energy and Industrial Strategy, if he will request that the Medical Research Council conducts an inquiry into the management of the PACE trial to ascertain whether any fraudulent activity has occurred.

Answer: Answered by: Joseph Johnson 28 November 2016

Queen Mary University of London, as the research organisation which held the award, is responsible for the management of the study, including the investigation of any concerns relating to research conduct and research integrity.

Whilst the Medical Research Council (MRC) was one of the funders of the PACE trial, the responsibility for the management of the trial rested with the host research institution, Queen Mary University of London (QMUL). This responsibility included oversight of the trial and the investigation of any well-founded allegations of misconduct that are brought to its attention. As part of this oversight, in accordance with MRC guidance on best practice, a trial steering committee was set up and supported by various sub-groups, including a data monitoring committee. The MRC was an observer on the trial steering committee.

Anyone wishing to raise concerns to over the conduct of individual researchers or research programmes is advised to contact QMUL in the first instance to allow the University to investigate appropriately. It would be inappropriate for BEIS to intervene in such investigations or to impose sanctions against researchers.

Question: 54266 Asked on: 22 November 2016

Department for Business, Energy and Industrial Strategy

Chronic Fatigue Syndrome: Research

To ask the Secretary of State for Business, Energy and Industrial Strategy, if he will prevent the PACE trial researchers from being given further public research funding until an inquiry into possible fraudulent activity into the PACE trial has been conducted.

Answer: Answered by: Joseph Johnson 28 November 2016

Queen Mary University of London, as the research organisation which held the award, is responsible for the management of the study, including the investigation of any concerns relating to research conduct and research integrity.

Whilst the Medical Research Council (MRC) was one of the funders of the PACE trial, the responsibility for the management of the trial rested with the host research institution, Queen Mary University of London (QMUL). This responsibility included oversight of the trial and the investigation of any well-founded allegations of misconduct that are brought to its attention. As part of this oversight, in accordance with MRC guidance on best practice, a trial steering committee was set up and supported by various sub-groups, including a data monitoring committee. The MRC was an observer on the trial steering committee.

Anyone wishing to raise concerns to over the conduct of individual researchers or research programmes is advised to contact QMUL in the first instance to allow the University to investigate appropriately. It would be inappropriate for BEIS to intervene in such investigations or to impose sanctions against researchers.

Question: 54267 Asked on: 22 November 2016

Department of Health

Chronic Fatigue Syndrome

To ask the Secretary of State for Health, if he will institute a revision of NICE guidelines for chronic fatigue syndrome/myalgic encephalopathy.

Answer: Answered by: Nicola Blackwood 25 November 2016

I refer the hon. Member to the Answer I gave on 23 November 2016 to his Question 53645.

Grouped Questions: 54265

Question: 54265 Asked on: 22 November 2016
Department of Health
Chronic Fatigue Syndrome: Medical Treatments
To ask the Secretary of State for Health, if he will remove CBT and GET from the list of treatments for ME patients.
Answer: Answered by: Nicola Blackwood 25 November 2016
I refer the hon. Member to the Answer I gave on 23 November 2016 to his Question 53645.

Question: 54245 Asked on: 17 November 2016
Department of Health
Chronic Fatigue Syndrome
To ask the Secretary of State for Health, with reference to the PACE trial, Pacing, graded Activity and Cognitive Behaviour Therapy, if he will ask NICE and the NHS to revise their approach to treating myalgic encephalomyelitis to removing references to Cognitive Behaviour Therapy and Graded Exercise Therapy.
Answer: Answered by: Nicola Blackwood 23 November 2016
The National Institute for Health and Care Excellence (NICE) is an independent body and is responsible for ensuring that its guidance remains up to date. NICE has advised that it has brought forward the next review date for its guidance on the diagnosis and management of chronic fatigue syndrome/myalgic encephalomyelitis from 2019 to 2017 to coincide with the expected publication of relevant new evidence.
NICE's aim is to make a decision on whether an update of the

SCIENCE, POLITICS, …….and ME

> guideline is required by the end of 2017.

The answers to these questions illustrate a fundamental issue in our system whereby ministers are unwilling to tackle any problems seen to be difficult – and so deny patients adequate protection against further deleterious research being funded and carried out.

The WHO International Classification of Diseases[69] has defined ME under the Neurological code G.93.3 some years ago but they have done little since. At one time the WHO made malaria, women's and children's health, venereal diseases, nutrition and environmental sanitation to be their priorities. New diseases, like AIDS, were added at a later period. It is time to address ME. Their success with smallpox and polio is well known. WHO interventions in emergencies and non-emergencies cover the globe. There are other offshoots of the UN, e.g. UNICEF, which focus on specific health issues with sectors of the world's population. They hold designated days to draw attention to World Autism Awareness, Mental Health, and Diabetes.

Yet as we write it seems that the WHO is in a process of revising the International Classification of Diseases (ICD) codes. Preliminary draft revisions of the ICD11 beta draft does not even show ME or CFS.

Whether this has underlying political motives is open to debate.

But it raises questions for patients, their families, carers, physicians, researchers and others as to whether Science, Politics and ME will ever be separated.

What is required is the initiation of a large education programme for general practitioners, nurses and other professionals as we are

---

[69] http://www.who.int/classifications/icd/en/

now witnessing with dementia.

In London in 2016 a group from USA, Europe and New Zealand was formed to look a medical education.

The European ME Alliance (EMEA) – a collaborating organisation composed of European patient groups and charities – is actively lobbying at the European level and engaging with the EU to bring about change.

Only a political consensus is going to break down the prejudices and control by an apparent elite. A recent book on ME does not even mention political influence as if it did not matter. Tell that to those who have borne the stigmatisation of AIDS, Autism, dementia etc.

The definition of ME, or lack of it, can no longer be an excuse for doing nothing. The history of medicine shows clearly how non-fashionable illnesses can move onto the centre stage.

We believe that the public must retain control of these discussions and will be the key players. As political parties are finding out, there can be almost overnight an overturn of the old order of politics e.g. Corbyn in the UK and Saunders and Trump in the USA. We believe this will happen too in European countries and elsewhere. We have seen the beginnings in Spain, Greece and Scotland. The mood is changing and medicine and science must move with it. For too long learned scientists have selected a pool of experts to give 'the line' and to promote with media support the thinking around subjects like ME. We won't say more about the media because it is almost an axiom in the Western world that they resist change and with very few notable exceptions play it 'safe', or are heavily biased in support of certain lobbies. The phone-hacking scandals of recent years show how the establishment controls the outcome and retain their power in the media, even after intensive inquiries and media coverage. The Jimmy Saville affair demonstrates how the establishment covers up when confronted with something it does not wish to discuss – at the expense of the public and the victims.

How do we involve the public?

Some charities and some prominent individuals have made huge inroads as far as informing the public of the problems with ME – such as Professor Malcolm Hooper, Countess of Mar and Margaret Williams. Yet people still suffer and as our interviews show ME is, as they say, a Cinderella subject!

Denying it exists and recommending treatments which have limited or deleterious effects on the patient (CBT and GET etc.) only perpetuates the myth that ME is not a real disease and this is then believed by the masses. The public becomes cynical, and if it doesn't affect them or their nearest and dearest, they simply shut off. They are seduced with the belief that there is no money at a time of austerity.

However, we need only mention the millions spent on IT programmes that have failed in Scotland and England to show that this is a knee-jerk reaction.

Millions were also found for proton therapy for cancer patients with brain tumours after a massive media publicity campaign in 2014 over a young boy, Ashya King, whose parents took him to Europe for the treatment that was not available in the UK.

Meanwhile grey figures in local commissioning groups and government funded health bodies continue to allocate monies to their 'priorities'. People are duped into thinking that money is the answer when clearly there are serious management problems of competence and attempts at imposing schemes where there is no evidence of success. Sometimes even we are told the 'new idea' has been imported from the USA where it works. Here the evidence is often scanty. Money has and is seriously wasted on IT schemes in the health service, PFI schemes which drain the health service of resources, changes to practitioners' contracts and many more could be mentioned. Attempts to take on these major problems are simply rejected and long term solutions ignored.

The recent rather diluted response of staff on the issues is hopefully only the tip of the iceberg. We often think those who power the policies in the NHS encourage a little revolt or two since it continues to drive the NHS into the avaricious hands of the privateers.

There are, then, the beginnings of a new network of scientists in the field of ME research. A new consortium is needed, not like the MRC collaboration, but a real one involving grass-roots scientists and patient groups with a mission to collaborate jointly across boundaries. We saw the beginnings in London recently with the announcement of collaborative work across Europe with individual scientists and patient groups who are not part of the government 'initiatives' drawn up by the Medical Research Council.

It is called EMERG (European ME Research Group) and its main objective across Europe is to establish a sustainable network of researchers working on ME. Before the recent inaugural EMERG meeting a subgroup of members had applied a second time for an EU COST (European Cooperation in Science and Technology) grant for ME infrastructure (meetings, working groups etc.) and this had been successful. These European initiatives will be built on principles of multidisciplinarity, patient and stakeholder involvement, strategic coordination with multiple sectors (researchers, clinicians, and industry looking for translational platforms for new treatment development), attraction of early career investigators, and contribute to the fostering of international cooperation.

Today in the Western world too many charities and patient organisations become corporate bodies more concerned with fund raising and structures or governance than they need be. They forget their purpose and become weighed down with issues that are outside their original aims. A programme for research money becomes a way of using money to appoint administrators or the one off projects that are not part of the whole picture nor part of the problem to provide better support for the patient. Some charities therefore seem to exist simply for the sake of existing.

A major coup was achieved at the Invest in ME Research London 2016 Colloquium and Conference when Professor Ron Davis of Stanford joined the fray and outlined the Big Data approach to the problem. This points to another way forward in terms of those engaged in research. The door for collaboration on a global scale seems to be open but there are doubters in the USA who have heard it all before. Many avenues of biomedical research were discussed and he illustrated how the 'team' would draw it together and concentrate on what 'might work'. At the same meeting Dr Vickie Whittemore from the NIH in Bethesda, Washington made it absolutely clear how grant requests were to be welcomed from across Europe. She intervened several times to emphasise how joint working was the way forward. She pointed out too how various agencies (like the ones involved in the Incline Village saga) needed to collaborate and communicate with each other and how Lupus had large-scale investment for research compared with ME. The huge input of resources into the Human Genome Project involving such collaboration and how the investment of further resources and money was essential. It was time to stop hiding behind Congress (or by implication the UK government) and take up the cudgels for biomedical research into ME.

The Nobel Prize winner, Jim Watson in the USA, was

collaborating with Professor Davis and had asked 2 questions:

How many people are affected and how much is being invested?

Put my name forward for the Board was his reply.

Compare this with the answer from the current minister in the UK who when asked by an MP the same questions, replied -

'We do not know'.

Diseases are often sold to the public as mere 'hysteria' as was ME or the way AIDS was sold as the 'gay disease', accompanied by the stories of it being transmitted from indulgence in sexual behaviour with animals. The media loves these types of stories and delight in easy explanations. The charities and other groups must take on the media and publish the views of prominent people, such as the Norwegian Prime Minister, and those affected in the population with the odd celebrity thrown in.

The President of the Royal Society of Psychiatrists, Sir Simon Wessely, turned up in the junior hospital doctors' dispute in the UK in 2016 to say 'The loss of anything other than a tiny minority of these junior doctors will be a substantial loss to the National Health Service.' This is the quote for quote's sake and adds nothing to the problems with the lessening of morale in the workplace.

The quote was a reference to the 7168 doctors trained for £250,000 each to undergo a 2-year training course following graduation. Some take jobs in higher education, some take a career break, others elect to work as a locum. There was much dissatisfaction amongst these young doctors and some members of the public wondered about their commitment, especially after a series of strikes that are still ongoing. This does not bode well for the future of the NHS.

Whilst ME is not a part of their training the situation does not lend much hope for their involvement with less fashionable illnesses, like ME, at least as far as the NHS is concerned. It is even less likely that researchers will emerge from science or medicine to further our understanding of ME, given the perverse publicity. Unless a new contract is agreed, despite government pressures, there will be gaps in the workforce of GPs that will affect the treatment and safety of patients.

Whilst Professor Wessely has publicly given up on ME research, he commented out of the blue and very soon after, to a Radio Norfolk show a few years ago, when the author, Ian Gibson, referred to the opposition to ME by the medical profession. His name often came up in discussions with university Heads of School (Deans) in Norwich who were resisting our activities for biomedical research into ME at UEA in Norwich. This was in the face of academic research and publications that continued to undermine the biopsychosocial approach and most particularly the PACE trial that promoted GET and CBT therapies.

A paper published in the Journal of Neurology and Neurobiology in March 2016 goes further to debunk the stories surrounding the results of the PACE trial:

46% of patients reported an increase in ME symptoms, 31% reported musculoskeletal and 19% reported neurological adverse events. Therefore, the proportion negatively affected by CBT and GET would be between 46% and 96.

Medication with such high rates of adverse events would be withdrawn with immediate effect. There was no difference in long-term outcomes between adaptive pacing therapy, CBT, GET and specialist medical care, and none of them were effective, invalidating the biopsychosocial model and use of CBT and GET for ME/CFS.[70]

Sten Helmfrid has gone even further in his article published in the influential Swedish journal Socialmedicinsk tidskrift [71] where he states -

> 'There is no scientific support for the treatment model used by the Oxford school, and its proponents have caused confusion by using inaccurate terms in the scientific literature and by presenting exaggerated claims. In science, a theory or a model is a description of the mechanisms behind a phenomenon. (A model should not be confused with a treatment model, which is merely a flow chart for the therapeutic efforts.) If a theory, model or other scientific proposition does not yet have empirical support, it is called a hypothesis. The interventions with cognitive behavioral therapy and graded exercise therapy are based on a hypothesis that the disease is perpetuated by avoidance behavior and that symptoms are caused by a lack of fitness. Although the Oxford school have not described any underlying mechanisms, nor presented any evidence for the presumed causation, they refer to their hypotheses either as theories or models. This gives the impression of scientific support, which in fact does not exist.
>
> When the hypotheses of the Oxford school first were introduced, the authors described their ideas with an analogy. They accepted that infections often are triggers for ME/CFS, but they pointed out that for example in a hit-and-run accident, pursuing the guilty party is not necessary in order to get

---

[70] Vink M (2016) The PACE Trial Invalidates the Use of Cognitive Behavioral and Graded Exercise Therapy in Myalgic Encephalomyelitis/Chronic Fatigue Syndrome: A Review. Journal of Neurobiology 2(3): doi http://dx.doi.org/10.16966/2379--7150.124

[71] *Socialmedicinsk tidskrift* [reference Helmfrid S. Studier av kognitiv beteendeterapi och gradvis ökad träning vid ME/CFS är missvisande. Soc Med Tidskr. 2016;93(4):433–44.]

started with the rehabilitation of the victim. Similarly, it is not necessary to know what triggered ME/CFS in the first place. The analogy misses an important point. When victims of a traffic accident are rehabilitated, doctors must know what injuries they have sustained—fractures require different therapies than burns—and when ME/CFS is treated, the rehabilitation strategy must resonate with the true perpetuating factors. The hit-and-run traffic analogy gives no hint as to whether the proposed strategy really works. '

We now have a tremendous opportunity to take the approach to treatment of ME into new pastures. We must forget the forlorn debates of what it is or is not in terms of general symptoms like fatigue. It is the patient who needs to be central in the opportunities for new research. The tiresome arguments and awaiting drug companies to take up the issue are irrelevant.

As Invest in ME Research has shown, you can crowd fund and raise support from the people involved with ME and initiate new directions for research. A recent conference on dementia that one of the authors attended heard of lack of research money. This was in front of a large, committed audience of patients, carers, charities, academics, care homes and administrators of the many health bodies. A concerted campaign amongst them could have set the ball rolling. Much as we agree that the state should fund the research, care and treatments, we cannot wait for 3rd rate politicians to mouth their concern and talk of 'unacceptability'. It is time to question our age-old approaches to the scientific understanding of a disease. A biomarker as a 'unit cause' is to be desired but it may be more complex as we find with some cancers. There may be several genetic events and complex relationships with environmental effects and in epigenetics that complicate simplistic explanations.

Let us start by educating doctors and medical students of the latest developments regarding biomedical research into ME until our researchers advance our understanding sufficiently to develop treatments.

Now is the time to encourage patient groups to take up the challenges. It is time to question those who run our health services and, if necessary, replace them with people who know what they are talking about. We need an educational initiative on a global basis and here the UN can help. We well remember the Blair government putting money into care and mental health treatments. It either didn't get sent, or got lost in the bureaucratic system that decided to pay off debts first before initiating new policies. It is time to have politicians and civil servants on the end of questioning to explain the gaps in ME research and treatment. Select Committees of Parliament and Inquiries are only one way to raise the issues but will need international initiatives. It simply won't happen if we leave it to each country.

There is hope now that this will occur if the NIH really do step up and support a strategy of biomedical research into this disease.

Research will inevitably follow on with some interesting answers but it must learn from past mistakes where far too much concentration has been placed on policies supporting the BPS model.

Prior to the publication of the 2002 CMO report into ME the psychiatrists walked out – but they continued to get all the funding for their biopsychosocial model. That must change as highlighted in the Gibson Inquiry.

A major investment of millions is needed to set up laboratories and research centres and hire both young and experienced staff. People are crying out for treatment. We are failing them and this must be righted. The time has passed for a blame culture and we must move on to doing better science and treating those who wish to 'have a life'.

At a recent meeting in Zurich of patient groups from 20 European countries to tackle the issues in the treatment of Multiple Sclerosis. Whilst it initially appeared there could be no agreement, as each country had its own priorities, it was decided that an early diagnosis of Multiple Sclerosis was universally required. This illustrates how agreements can be reached when people of the same concerns meet and argue for a uniform requirement to improve lives of patients with MS. It also shows that in different European countries agreement on joint research programmes and treatments can become a major campaign.

Far from leaving the European union, we should in the UK be attempting to get agreements which can be followed for patients and which break down the postcode lottery within and between countries. Working for a uniform programme would have tremendous benefits as it did for cancer treatments in the UK.

For ME this is exactly what the European ME Alliance (EMEA) has agreed to do – sharing common principles and working toward similar aims in each member countries as well as lobbying at European level in the European Parliament.

So the seeds for hope are there.

As a parting shot let us repeat the pledges for publication and a pledge card which Ian Gibson outlined at the 2016 conference in London. They make good targets and have worked in focussing attention on key issues as in the 1998 cancer programme (outlined in the All Party Cancer Group), which were successful then, and could be again:

(i) Development of strong European, International scientific collaborations

(ii) Education programmes about ME on a local, national and international level

(iii) Vast increases in research funding, especially in the molecular and physiological arenas

(iv) A Centre of Excellence for ME in the UK/Europe involving research and treatment and leading to others around the world that can collaborate

(v) Equal access to diagnosis and treatment

Chapter 7 - Concluding Remarks

As this book goes to print the establishment media has been heralding a 'new' way of treating young people with ME/CFS. The trial of 700 under-18 year olds through the NHS FITNET Trial, University of Bristol, is described as having value for money compared with other treatments. The treatment is based on Activity Management using video conferencing. This may be more economical and accessible than the sparse clinical provision but it is a short sighted way of money saving rather than providing the resources for biological research and treatment to children and young people with ME/CFS.

The Trial, with NHS funding, began on 1 November and is expected, like the controversial and widely denigrated PACE Trial, to produce 'positive' results through its selective criteria and assessment methods.

Once again, it uses Cognitive Behavioural Therapy, a psychological tool, as its main source of treatment.

In light of the PACE Trial it appears incomprehensible as to why further funding should be given for research down this route.

Meanwhile in Norfolk a Centre of Excellence for biomedical research into ME is being established. Invest in ME Research is behind the initiative to create an international centre for scientific research into ME/CFS with 5 PhD students currently enrolled to carry out work in the dedicated laboratory. The research is carried out with collaboration across Europe, in particular with Haukeland University in Bergen where the original Rituximab Trial took place. The emphasis is on high quality biomedical research. With this new Centre being developed based on biomedical research and international collaboration, much of the conflict between psychological versus biomedical arguments could be resolved. This is the hope of many patients who have long been waiting for some definitive scientific research.

It is initiatives such as this which ought to command support as it can pave a new way of thinking to be brought in for science and thus avoid the terrible injustices being performed on citizens by corrupted policies and vested interests.

Compare the amount of media attention given to the above two proposals and one can clearly see what has been so wrong with the treatment of ME and what could be so right using a correct model for approaching the disease.

Perhaps the final paragraphs of this book should be from patients and carers.

The charity Invest in ME Research, run by volunteer patients and carers, voiced its concerns about past faults in official policy to ME and paths for future progress in its response to the NIH Pathways To Prevention (P2P) report [72]. The following is taken from the closing remarks from their report to the NIH – but the statements that could apply to all countries where policies toward ME have been influenced by politics instead of science –

> .... we hope our views are taken on board as this affects not only US citizens but everyone diagnosed with ME or CFS across the world.

> It does not help that research into ME/CFS has two opposite viewpoints and this document (*P2P report*) consequently tries to facilitate both.

---

[72] http://investinme.org/IIME-Newslet-1501-01.shtml

This is a major mistake and is contrary to any common sense.

It is illogical to do this and if the statement is made that ME/CFS is a physical disease then recommendations should follow logically from that statement.
If there are co-morbidities they should be dealt with in the same way as one would do with co-morbidities in MS, cancer or Parkinson's disease or any other disease.

We ....sincerely hope that this is not yet another paper exercise to keep the patient community seemingly happy whilst the authorities do nothing concrete to remedy the current situation.

It would be well for the NIH **NOT** to follow the UK example and repeat the mistakes and failures of the last generation where an insincere effort to change is portrayed as real progress but just results in wasted years.
The mediocrity in terms of provision of correct and up to date definitions and guidelines, scientific research and development of treatments and perception of ME is a direct result, and failure, of the policies of the past.
....
We believe future research into ME must be based on collaboration. But it would seem quite meaningless to base the strategy on those failed policies and directions of the past - which have served patients so poorly and caused such suffering.

> Research into ME needs a strategic approach - but it may be destined to fail completely by attempting to establish the way forward (based) on foundations which include so much of what has been wrong in the past.
>
> If we are seriously to have a way forward for proper research into ME then we need not just funding, but correctly defined cohorts, standardisation on diagnostic criteria and a collaborative of researchers who will not blur science with politics.

The NIH have a unique possibility to be bold, to fix this problem once and for all.

We therefore suggest the following –
We suggest that the NIH finally and totally abandon all links to the biopsychosocial model with regard to ME research funding.
We also suggest that instead of relying on alternative funding streams elsewhere that the NIH take responsibility themselves for ME/CFS.

We suggest that the NIH invest $50 million per year for the next five years in biomedical research into ME/CFS, and provide correct and current education into the disease which will, in turn, raise appropriate awareness.
This would mean an investment of $250 million over 5 years.
This amount will still be less than the documented annual cost of ME/CFS of $1 billion as noted in line 6.

This will create scores of biomedical research projects, lots of potential international collaboration, new ideas and new skills to enter the ME/CFS research area.

This will facilitate the harnessing of the full potential of academic and research institutes.

This will attract new, young researchers into the field of ME/CFS – this the charity has proven already with our B-Cell/rituximab project with UCL where a young researcher is drawn into this exciting area of research [21]

It will galvanise science and eventually form pockets of expertise which will create the centres of excellence for the future.

We suggest trying this for a 5-year period.
A yearly review of progress can inform every one of the status.

After 5 years of such funding a new conference/workshop/committee can be convened and progress can be examined.

This will provide the best chance possible for resolving this illness to the benefit of patients.

Our guess is that so much progress will have been made in research, in perception and possibly in treatments during that period that the money will be recouped with the added benefit of giving some people their lives back.

The stigma mentioned above – which is actually, in our opinion, just ignorant prejudice created by corrupt organisations and individuals - would be swept away.

$50 million per year is really not much.

After 5 years it will probably have so much momentum that it could carry on by itself through savings in welfare, through new discoveries and, yes, through private donations/funding
....

We invite the NIH .... to join our international collaboration effort to resolve this illness in a way that brings hope to patients, brings responsible and proper science to the research area and brings a raising of awareness that will obliterate the monstrous distortions about ME/CFS which have poisoned all chance of making progress in the last generation.

What needs to be emphasised to all – something that is rarely acknowledged and which we see ignored by almost every organisation – is the urgency of the need for action and change.

> This is urgent, lives are dependent on it – Treat it as being urgent!
> To make progress we need not mere words and a slow undeliberate action plan.
>
> Progress is a fine word – but change is its motivator

To progress this illness we need to make bold changes.

Invest in ME Research is a small charity with a BIG cause.
If such a small charity and its supporters can organise (twelve) international conferences with delegates from 20 countries, if it can organise (seven) biomedical research colloquiums attracting participants from top research organisations in a dozen countries, if it can initiate possibly the two most important research projects for ME in the UK then the NIH should be able to do far, far better – and in a far shorter period of time.

In the words of the charity's advisor Dr Ian Gibson –

"Things do not have to be the way they are – we can change things.".

Science, Politics …….and ME.

These have not been happy bedfellows for the last generation.

Whilst patients want nothing more than to regain their health, the science which should be available to help them achieve that objective has been thwarted by the politics of the establishment and those who retain influence at the highest levels.

This must change.

Appendix 1 - Programme of 11th Invest in ME Research International ME Conference 2016

We reproduce the programme of the scientists and carers, patients and non-patients, held in 2016 in London by Invest in ME Research (IiMER).

The 11th International Invest in ME Research Conference, London June 2016

The conference, chaired by the author, Dr Ian Gibson, brought together world experts in research into ME. The list of contributors for the 2016 conference is below:

- Dr Vicky Whittemore, Program Director Channels, Synapses and Circuits Cluster at NIH/NINDS and the leader of a Trans-NIH Working Group on ME/CFS, Bethesda, USA

- Dr Olli Polo, Chief, Department of Pulmonary Medicine, Tampere University Hospital, Tampere, Finland

- Professor Carmen Scheibenbogen, Deputy Director of the Institute of Medical Immunology, Charité, Berlin, Germany

- Dr Jo Cambridge, Professorial Research Associate, Division of Rheumatology, Department of Medicine, University College London, UK

- Mr Fane Mensah, PhD student, Division of Rheumatology, Department of Medicine at the University College London, UK

- Professor Tom Wileman, Professor of Infection & Immunity at the Norwich Medical School, and Director of the Biomedical Research Centre, University of East Anglia, Norwich, UK

- Professor Don Staines, Co-Director National Centre for Neuroimmunology & Emerging Diseases, Griffith Health Institute, Griffith University, QLD, Australia

- Professor Simon Carding, Professor of Mucosal Immunology/Research Leader Gut Health, Institute of Food Research, Norwich, UK

- Associate Professor Mady Hornig, Director Translational Research / Assoc. Professor Epidemiology, Center for Infection and Immunity (CII), Mailman School of Public Health, Columbia University, New York, USA

- Professor Maureen Hanson, Liberty Hyde Bailey Professor, Department of Molecular Biology & Genetics, Cornell University, Ithaca, NY, USA

- Professor Elisa Oltra, Professor of Cell and Molecular Biology at the Universidad Católica de Valencia - San Vicente Mártir, Valencia, Spain

- Professor James Baraniuk, Professor of Medicine, Georgetown University Medical Centre, Washington, D.C., USA

- Professor Ron Davis, Professor of Biochemistry & Genetics, Director of the Stanford Genome Technology Center, Stanford University, USA.

The proceedings of the 11th International Conference held in London on June 3, 2016 are available as a DVD at: http://www.investinme.eu/IIMEC11.shtml#dvd

Several important research papers have appeared in the past few months since conference. The first significant one comes from the group led by Professor Ron Davis. Headlined the 'Metabolic features of chronic fatigue syndrome', it appeared under the name Naviaux et al in the Journal, Proceedings of the National Academy of Sciences of the USA Vol. 113, 37. Interestingly, the work was funded by several private foundations and individuals. Pointing out the difficulty of diagnosis because of its many symptoms and the lack of a diagnostic laboratory test, the work resorts to looking at a significant number of ME patients who had what were called abnormalities in 20 metabolic pathways. The latter involved e.g. phospholipids, purine, cholesterol microbiome, riboflavin and mitochondrial metabolism. They concluded that despite the heterogeneity of factors leading to ME/CFS the metabolic response in patients was exactly the same, robust statistically with similarities to responses for environmental stress. This is a new way of analysing complex illnesses and sharply contrasts with DNA analysis and in this new way blood is analysed for chemicals, some 2000 or so metabolites. This approach, it is felt, represents the individual at the time of analysis – not ancestral relationship as in DNA analysis. Hopefully this might lead to actions preventing any one individual metabolic variation to restore the correct chemical balance. It clearly would serve as a marker utilising the study of each metabolic pathway variation. To sum up these changes, shown in the article, represent not just one causal agent or molecule but the effects of a confection of (particular) chemical changes in several pathways. This is a fresh way of thinking about an illness model which is appropriate for many illnesses which have been relegated to 'other' explanations or left on the shelf as being of no interest since a 'cure' is not something likely to be around the corner as a personalised treatment or as a diagnostic tool.

This new approach is called metabolomics. Substances can be above or below a mean and comparisons made with other body onslaughts. The conclusions of the research group EMERG (European ME Research Group) is that 'effective treatments for CFS/ME are likely to be achieved by careful attention to nutrition, metabolism, triggers, stressors or physical activity as part of an integrated biophysical system.

Other working proceeding from laboratories in Europe and indeed across the world involve the work of Marshall-Gradisnik and Don Staines in the Gold Coast of Australia with their work on the dysregulation of protein kinase gene expression in NK cells from ME/CFS patients.[73]

The Norwegian group are still working with others like Jo Cambridge in UCL laboratories in London but although their recent work does not at this stage bring significant advances they

---

[73] Anu Chacko, Donald R. Staines, Samantha C. Johnston and Sonya M. Marshall-Gradisnik. "Dysregulation of Protein Kinase Gene Expression in NK Cells from Chronic Fatigue Syndrome/Myalgic Encephalomyelitis Patients" **Gene Regulation and Systems Biology** 2016:10 85-93

are working tirelessly to understand the role of immunological responses to rituximab in the cell immune system. A new literature is emerging on the effects of the microbiome on the illness. At the same time new research is asking where the microbiome comes from in relation to evolution. In Norwich Wileman and Carding are questioning and researching the bacteriophages. They are looking at the possible directed destruction of microbes by the viruses thereby changing 'good' from 'bad' bacteria or vice-versa depending on the control of the bacteriophage populations and the conditions which change these populations.

Appendix 2 – UK Government Ministers of Health

Since CMO's Report of 2002 and onwards -

Alan Milburn (Labour) 11 October 1999 - 13 June 2003

John Reid (Labour) 13 June 2003 - 6 May 2005

Patricia Hewitt (Labour) 6 May 2005 - 27 June 2007

Alan Johnson (Labour) 28 June 2007 - 5 June 2009

Andy Burnham (Labour) 5 June 2009 - 1 May 2010

Andrew Lansley (Cons.) 11 May 2010 - 4 September 2012

Jeremy Hunt (Cons.) 4 September 2012 -

(current at time of publication)

Appendix 3 – References

- Boulton, N. (ed.) (2010) *Lost Voices from a Hidden Illness.* Wild Conversations Press

- Bristol University (2013), www.bris.ac.uk/news/2013/9741.html

- British Medical Journal (2013) *BMJ* 2013;347:f5731

- Centre for Welfare Reform, www.centreforwelfarereform.org

- Chacko A., Staines D.R., Johnston S.C. and Marshall-Gradisnik S.M. *Dysregulation of Protein Kinase Gene Expression in NK Cells from Chronic Fatigue Syndrome/Myalgic Encephalomyelitis Patients* in *Gene Regulation and Systems Biology* 2016:10 (85-93)

- Dimmock M and Lazell Fairman M (2015) *Thirty Years of Disdain: How HHS buried ME.* http://bit.ly/The_Burial_of_ME_Background

- Edwards, Jonathan et al (2015) *The Biological Challenge of ME/CFS.* European ME Research Group (EMERG) Meeting London 13th October 2015

- European ME Research Group Meeting (2016) http://www.investinme.org/em-index.shtml

- Fluge Ø, et al. (2015) B-Lymphocyte depletion in myalgic encephalopathy/chronic fatigue syndrome. An open-label phase II study with rituximab maintenance treatment. PLoS One, 2015 Jul 1; 10(7)

- Gibson I. (2006) The Gibson Enquiry Report – The Group on Scientific Research in Myalgic Encephalomyelitis. http://www.erythos.com/gibsonenquiry/Report.html

- Gibson I. (2007) Witness statement in support of the Judicial Review case of the NICE "CFS/ME" Guideline (CG53) online brought by ME patients: Re: Douglas Fraser & Kevin Short v NICE. HM Government, Case Number: CO/10408/2007.

- Goldstein, D. (2004) *Once upon a virus: AIDS legends and vernacular risk perception.* Logan, USA: Utah State University Press

- Hanley, Jesse L. and Deville, Nancy (2001) *Tired of Being Tired: Rescue, Repair, Rejuvenate.* Penguin: Puttnam.

- Hansard (1998) reference to the "*Wessely School*" in Hansard: Lords: 9th December 1998:1013

- Hare, David. *Why the Tory Project is Bust.* The Guardian, Tuesday 8 March 2016.

- Hawkes, Nigel (2011). 'Dangers of research into chronic fatigue syndrome'. BMJ 2011;342:d3780

- Heckenively K. and Mikovits J. (2014) Plague: One Scientist's Intrepid Search for the Truth about Human Retroviruses and Chronic Fatigue Syndrome (ME/CFS), Autism and Other Diseases. New York: Skyhorse Publishing, Inc.

- Hemispherx (2015). www.hemispherx.net and www.nasdaq.com/press-release/hemispherx-biopharma

- HM Government (2015) www.informationtribunal.gov.uk

- Hooper, M. 'Fatigue', *Biomedicine, Health & Behavior* 2016:4:3 (127-13).

- Institute of Medicine (2015) Committee on the Diagnostic Criteria for Myalgic Encephalomyelitis/Chronic Fatigue Syndrome, Board on the Health of Select Populations, *Beyond Myalgic Encephalomyelitis* Washington DC: National Academies Press (US).

- The 11th Revision of the International Classification of Diseases (ICD-11) http://www.who.int/classifications/icd/revision/en/

- Invest in ME Research, www.investinme.org

- Leslie, Mitch (2016) Fighting autoimmunity with immune cells' Science 14: 1 July, 2016

- Let's Do It For Me, www.ldifme.org

- McElroy, A. and Townsend, P. (2009) *Medical Anthropology in Ecological Perspective*. Colorado: Westview Press.

- MailOnline (2015) www.dailymail.co.uk/health/article-3292782: 28 October 2015

- Medical Research Council (2003) *New Research Directions for CFS/ME*.

- NHS (2015), www.nhs.uk/conditions/chronic-fatigue-syndrome

- Shakespeare, Tom, Watson N. and Alghaib O.A. (2016) Blaming the victim, all over again: Waddell and Aylward's biophyschosocial (BPS) model of disability in Critical Social Policy 2016, Vol 36:4 (1-20)

- Sheffield Hallam University (2003) http://news.bbc.co.uk/1/hi/health/3014341.stm

- Silberman, Steve (2015) Neurotribes: The Legacy of Autism and How to Think Smarter About People Who Think Differently. London: Allen and Unwin.

- Sontag S. (1977) *Illness as Metaphor*. Toronto: McGraw-Hill Ryerson

- Speight, Nigel (2012). http://voicesfromtheshadowsfilm.co.uk/nigel-speight-me-handout

- The Nursing Times 'Parliamentary Group hits out at lack of support for ME' March, 2010

- The Telegraph online, www.telegraph.co.uk

- The Guardian online www.theguardian.co.uk

- Turner, D. and Gibson I. (2013) *Best When We Are Labour?* Brighton: Pen Press Publications.

- Twisk, F.N. (2016) Replacing Myalgic Encephalomyelitis and Chronic Fatigue Syndrome with Systemic Exercise Intolerance Disease Is Not the Way forward. *Diagnostics* 2016:6, 10.

- Waddell G. and Aylward M. (2005) *Models of Sickness and Disability applied to common health problems.* Centre for Psychosocial and Disability Research, School of Medicine, University of Cardiff.

- Wallace, Anthony (1972) *Mental Illness, Biology and Culture* in Psychological Anthropology pp362-402.

- Vink M. The PACE Trial Invalidates the Use of Cognitive Behavioral and Graded Exercise Therapy in Myalgic Encephalomyelitis/Chronic Fatigue Syndrome: A Review. Journal of Neurobiology, 2016: 2 (3)

- Virology (2015) Trial by Error: The Troubling Case of the PACE Chronic Fatigue Syndrome Study. www.virology.ws/2015/10/21/trial-by-error-i

Printed in Great Britain
by Amazon